PRAISE FOR URBAN TANTRA

"Any book on Tantra that begins by describing a professional lap dance as a divine sexual experience is one I will definitely read. Written with wit and humor, Barbara's *Urban Tantra* keeps sex real, and, best of all, the rituals are fun."

—Betty Dodson, PhD, author of *Sex for One* and *Orgasms for Two*

"If you ever thought Tantra wasn't for you—too foreign or gimmicky or New Agey, or not edgy enough for your radical sex explorations—Barbara Carrellas will cure you of all misconceptions and bring you an Urban Tantra to unite your sex, your spirit, your erotic wanderlust, your edge."

—Carol Queen, author of *Real Live Nude Girl*

"*Urban Tantra* offers a daring, delicious, profound, courageous, and altogether magical celebration that will teach us all to dance to the rhythms of the universe. Barbara Carrellas has written the ultimate how-to book that unites sex with spirit, healing with philosophy, and the animating force of the cosmos with each and every one of us. So if you'd like to live your sex life on a galactic scale, you must read this book!"

—Dossie Easton, coauthor of *The Ethical Slut*

"Everyone needs to rejoice in their own sexuality, and Barbara shows us how in this very informative, easy-to-use book. It would be nice to practice Tantra in a lovely remote garden or high atop a mountain, but the reality is that in today's world many of us don't have that luxury. Barbara demonstrates that it doesn't matter where you practice, as long as you're conscious when you do. Now, let go and enjoy *Urban Tantra*."

—Louise Hay, author of *You Can Heal Your Life* and *Empowering Women*

"*Urban Tantra* is a courageous book by Barbara Carrellas, one of the pioneers in contemporary American Tantra. This engaging and comprehensive guide includes numerous powerful exercises as well as moving personal anecdotes that reveal how the conscious exploration and embrace of sexuality can function as a tool for transformation."

—Mark A. Michaels (Swami Umeshanand Saraswati) and Patricia Johnson (Devi Veenanand), authors of *The Essence of Tantric Sexuality*

"Barbara Carrellas, whose Urban Tantric sex workshops combine Eastern sex techniques with the postmodern methods of SM practitioners, is a trailblazer."

—Tristan Taormino, *The Village Voice*

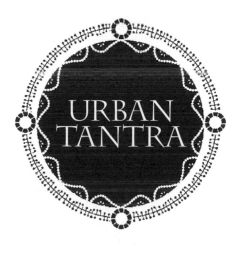

URBAN
TANTRA

URBAN TANTRA

sacred sex *for the* twenty-first century

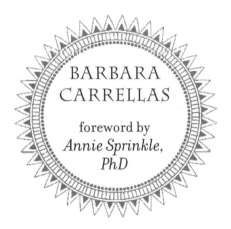

BARBARA
CARRELLAS

foreword by
Annie Sprinkle,
PhD

CELESTIAL ARTS
Berkeley | Toronto

Celestial Arts
PO Box 7123
Berkeley, California 94707
www.tenspeed.com

Distributed in Australia by Simon and Schuster Australia, in Canada by Ten Speed Press Canada, in New Zealand by Southern Publishers Group, in South Africa by Real Books, and in the United Kingdom and Europe by Publishers Group UK.

Book design by Kate Basart/Union Pageworks

The poem on the oppisite page is paraphrased from Guillaume Apollinaire.

Quotation on page 18 excerpted from *The Book of Secrets* by Osho. Copyright © 1974 by Osho International Foundation, Switzerland. www.osho.com. All rights reserved. Reprinted with permission.

Library of Congress Cataloging-in-Publication Data
Carrellas, Barbara.
    Urban tantra : sacred sex for the twenty-first century / Barbara Carrellas.
       p. cm.
    Includes bibliographical references and index.
    ISBN-13: 978-1-58761-290-9
    ISBN-10: 1-58761-290-9
    1. Sex. 2. Tantrism. 3. Sex instruction. I. Title.
    HQ23.C38 2007
    306.77—dc22
           2006100430

First printing, 2007
Printed in the United States of America

1 2 3 4 5 6 7 8 9 10 — 11 10 09 08 07

Come to the edge, she said.
No, I will fall.
Come to the edge.
No, it's too high.
Come to the edge.
I came
she pushed
and I flew.

This book is dedicated to
Louise L. Hay
&
Patricia M. Neilson

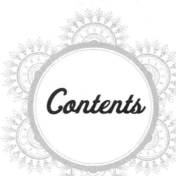

Contents

Acknowledgments

This book was first imagined several years ago in my warm and wild sex and spirituality workshops in Australia. It has taken the love and support of many people to take *Urban Tantra* off the massage table and put it on the page.

To my partner in love, art, and life, Kate Bornstein: Thank you for your unwavering belief in me and in the importance of this book. Thank you for the inspiration and encouragement to go far beyond the scope of my original idea. Thank you for reading every chapter of this book over and over again. Thank you for loving me.

To Chester Mainard: Thank you for giving me a language for bodies and pleasure. You are the finest teacher I have ever met, and teaching in partnership with you was one of the greatest thrills of my life. I have tried to capture the spirit of your teachings in *Urban Tantra*. I will love you forever.

To Louise L. Hay: Thank you for your unconditional love, for your continuing delight in my more extreme diversions, and for always being there when I need a good cry, a good laugh, or a good zing. Thank you especially for the intensity of your support during the final stages of this book.

Thanks to my sister-of-the heart, Annie Sprinkle, who held my hand as I dove into the deep end of sex and has been my dearest friend ever since. Thanks also to the other ladies of Club 90: Veronica Hart, Gloria Leonard, Candida Royalle, and Veronica Vera, who have encouraged me every step of the way. Special thanks to Linda Montano, who has provided me with spiritual guidance and art/life counseling for so many years.

I have learned so much from my friends and colleagues: Lily Burana, Kutira Decosterd, Betty Dodson, Raelyn Gallina, Lynda Gayle, Jwala, Robert Lawrence, Christiane Northrup, Carol Queen, Pat Sinatra, and especially Joseph Kramer. I am eternally grateful not only for what you have taught me, but also for allowing me to fold bits of your brilliance into this book.

It is much easier to explore sex in a country founded by convicts than one founded by puritans. My deepest thanks to my Australian national workshop coordinator and best mate, Hayley Caspers. Thanks to my brave and wise regional presenters, Margie Fischer, Sue Marley, Kirien Withers, Di Alexander, Alka, and Joanne Baker. The success of my workshops was in large part due to the physical, emotional, and psychic support of Catherine Carter, Steve Cairnduff, Heather Croall, Cyndi Darnell, Lianna

Gailand, Diana Haigh, Laura-Doe Harris, Debra Kaplan, Peter Masters, Jenny Navaro, Alison Partridge, Justine Watson, and norrie m⊕y welby, among others.

Thank you to my literary agent, Malaga Baldi, for your total devotion to and belief in this book. With your help, it has evolved into everything I imagined, and more.

Huge hugs of enthusiastic ecstasy to Colleen Coover, who created the perfect illustrations for *Urban Tantra*.

Gobs of gratitude to Celestial Arts, who helped heal the wounds of a past publishing nightmare with their respect, enthusiasm, and love, and particularly to my editor, Brie Mazurek. Brie, you are a star. Thanks also to Mark Rhysberger and Felice Newman for editorial help on an earlier version of the manuscript.

It's true—there are no people like show people. Thanks to James M. Nederlander, Herschel Waxman, and Jim Boese of the Nederlander Organization, and to the crew and staff of the Brooks Atkinson Theatre, who not only tolerated my frequent author's angst, but supported me with good humor and good cheer throughout the process. Most especially, my deepest thanks and love to Marilyn S. Miller, who covered countless performances for me so I could write. Bravo, all.

I am very grateful to Tristan Taormino for her ongoing support of my work as well as for her part in the creation of Dark Odyssey, a biannual sexual/spiritual retreat, where I have been inspired by so many erotic pioneers. Thanks especially to Anton, Susan Benner, Blair, Sir C, Colten Tognazzini, femcar, Bridgett Harrington, kate and David, Lolita, Major, and puppy for their wisdom and friendship. Extra special thanks to Tantric authors and teachers Mark Michaels and Patricia Johnson for their inspiration and camaraderie.

My gratitude to Mary Wallach and Rod DeJong, who cared for my emotional and physical bodies while I wrote, and to Osho, who continues to care for my soul.

Thanks to family members and friends: Matt Ainsworth, Lynn Birks and Judith Wit, Frances, Gizmo, Goose, Chele Graham, P. Kitty, Sara Miriam, Mollyanna, Patricia C. Lee, Patricia Neilson, Daniel Peralta, Beverly Petty, Kaylynn Raschke and Alexis Hurkman, and Ron Tillinghast, who gave me the space and opportunity to hide, scream, imagine, rage, howl, and giggle throughout the writing process.

To all the participants of my workshops for the past many years and to everyone at a play party, ritual, or erotic retreat who has ever blown me away with their honesty, passion, wisdom, courage, and creativity, thank you. You have inspired me and kept me on my path. This book is not only for you, it's also partially by you.

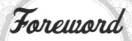

Foreword

BY ANNIE SPRINKLE, PhD

Barbara Carrellas asked me to write the foreword to her book, she said, because "we walked so much of this path together." This is true. We traveled thousands of miles, hand in hand (and hand elsewhere too), in search of the Holy Grail that was to become *Urban Tantra*. We followed our muses and used our sexualities to guide us toward wisdom and enlightenment.

Our adventure began in New York City in the mid-1980s, before *Sex in the City*, before Disney took over the delightfully sleazy Times Square, before there were Tantra workshops in every major city. Barbara was a mild-mannered Broadway theater manager, and I was an excruciatingly shy, insecure teenager who had faced her fears of men and sex and became Annie Sprinkle, proud prostitute and pioneering porn-star performance artist.

We met at a large support group called the New York Healing Circle during the "sex=death" years, when AIDS was out of control. Barbara was a recovering Catholic who was horribly squeamish about religion. I had been raised Unitarian/atheist, and I struggled with suddenly becoming interested in God/dess and spirituality. It took the deaths of our close friends and lovers to put us on what was to become a life-enhancing spiritual path.

Barbara and I hit it off immediately. We had a brief sexual relationship, which quickly evolved into a deep friendship. Barbara was already more sexually experienced and sex-positive than most folks. She taught me about my G-spot (thanks, Barb). But she was also inexperienced in some ways, and I thought she would just dip her toe into the "sex community" waters and then go back to a more straight-and-narrow path.

But instead, she got out there and started to learn everything she could about sexuality, gathering experience through excess. Together, we went to orgies, BDSM clubs, Times Square peep show palaces, and transsexual and hermaphrodite parties and tried it all with lots of people. Barbara even appeared in some innovative arty sex films, including two that I directed, and several HBO *Real Sex* segments. Barbara did it *all*, with class and great integrity.

At some point we started taking Tantra workshops from the small handful of Tantra teachers around back then. Originally, we were drawn to Tantra because it seemed to embrace everything: sexuality, passion, BDSM, fetish, piercing, sacred prostitutes, fisting—you name it. But most of the workshops seemed a little bit silly and too woo-woo for our tastes. We didn't jive with the all-white, middle-aged, strictly hetero-sexual couple-oriented, New Age Tantra thing, and we ran into some trouble, as we were always the only queer, edgy, freaky folks there. We were judged by what we were interested in and told, "That's not Tantra."

But the techniques we learned and the intentionality of Tantra resonated with us. When we learned about ecstasy breathing, we had some absolutely electrifying experiences with full-body energy orgasms, which were like chakra enemas, shamanic journeys, and religious experiences all rolled into one. Learning these relatively simple, ancient techniques changed the way we viewed and experienced sex and changed our lives forever.

We were so enthusiastic about what we were experiencing that we naturally wanted to share it with our friends and communities. We hit the road and started facilitating sexuality workshops together, learning more through teaching. Our "Sacred Sex," "Fun with Breath and Energy Orgasms," "Erotic Massage," and "Sluts and Goddesses" workshops were completely Tantric in spirit but quite different from traditional Tantric workshops. They included not just chanting, energy work, and meditation, but also sometimes BDSM, gender play, corsets, fetishes, whore/slut/witch archetypes, and more. Many of the wonderful people who came gave us heartfelt, occasionally teary, feedback about how they were liberated or how their lives were changed for the better because of something they learned. Many workshop participants inadvertently gave us some new key piece of information or new experience, deepening our own personal exploration.

Tantra provided a way for us to continue on a sexual journey and get our spiritual needs met, while giving us ways to cope with all the death and disease around us. Barbara and I felt like we were reclaiming sex from a messed-up, sexually dysfunctional, judgmental, and ignorant culture. It became our public service, our labor of love, our mission in life, to use sexuality to generate healing, transcendental, enriching experiences.

After many years of learning, working, and traveling together, we came to a fork in the road. I moved out of Manhattan to California. We both started teaching new workshops on our own. Barbara taught in Australia, often with the extremely gifted and enlightened teacher Chester Mainard. Then, later, she taught with Kate Bornstein, the visionary author, performer, activist, and "transgender outlaw." Being with Kate, Barbara learned a whole lot more about what it was to be truly queer, to not fit in, to be differently gendered. They taught workshops that reached a new, even more diverse audience looking for transformative experiences that fit their personalities and lifestyles.

Barbara continued the journey, discovering and creating new things at every turn, gathering what would become her own unique creation: a fresh, new, inclusive, smart, hip, bold, and very fun version of Tantra. I'm absolutely thrilled that people everywhere will get to revel in Barbara's wit and wisdom through this book's pages. *Urban Tantra* gives me hope that the world will become a more sexually satisfied, ecstatic, enlightened, and inclusive place.

Fellow traveler, as you now begin your journey, know that you are welcome here, whether you and/or your partner are inexperienced or experienced, young or old, differently abled or differently bodied, pierced or tattooed, interested in kink or not. It doesn't matter where you live, who you are, or what you do. You belong here. Barbara thinks you are perfect and sexy as you are, and she will teach you delightful, yummy new things to help you live your life ever more deliciously and meaningfully.

Now, I will leave you with this Urban Tantra mantra:

> *Om shanti panty*
> *Ha hari hairy*
> *Tit pat tooshie*
> *Just say ya ya yaaaaaa*
> *Taxi sat samosa*
> *Va va voom voom*
> *Jaya juicy ju ju*
> *Thy cum be yum*
> *Oh ma ma me-ah*
> *Nookie nir-va-na*
> *Yum yum yum*
> *Om. Welcome home. Om.*

Prelude

THE TEMPLE OF THE SACRED LAP DANCE, OR ECSTASY IS WHERE YOU FIND IT

August in New York is legendary for its soupy heat. Steam swirls up out of the subway gratings into the still, humid air and holds in an uneasy embrace everyone who can't escape to the swank beaches of Long Island and the Jersey Shore.

New York's financial district is even more claustrophobic in the August heat than most places in the city. The narrow streets and toweringly tall buildings prevent even the tiniest breath of cool air from finding you. In 1992, long before anyone could imagine that this neighborhood would ever be called Ground Zero, young financial whizzes not yet successful enough to spend these dog days in cooler climes dashed from air-conditioned tower to air-conditioned tower in their suits and ties. The mere sight of these tightly buttoned beings in the heat of the downtown streets made me gasp for air. The financial district was not a part of town I frequented, but I was going where the money was: I'd packed my best black lace bra and most expensive garter belt and G-string. The extra-long black stockings that completed my outfit were not expensive. Lap dancing is a sure way to go through several pairs in a single shift.

I'd only done lap dancing once before, but I'd learned fast. One, wear stockings; they hold the cash more securely than garters. That way you can give all your attention to the customer on whose lap you are gyrating, which in turn leads to a longer dance and more tips. Plus, stockings make your legs look longer and more alluring. Two, pick a persona that works for you and stick with it. In this club, I am "Alexandra," a high-class, uptown call girl type. A cool, sophisticated-looking blonde is unique in this dark, seedy place. We all base our personas on sexual stereotypes. The Latina women I work with favor the Charo, coochie-coochie look. The black women favor *Uptown Saturday Night*. The few white women who work at the Harmony favor a sporty, well-toned, athletic look. Alexandra is an oddity here, and that's always a plus in this business. Her what-if-Grace-Kelly-were-a-hooker quality appeals to a sizable clientele in this part of town.

I am working at the Harmony Burlesque because I need money—fast. My girlfriend is in Australia looking after her sick mum and has invited me to join her for a couple of weeks. She has even sent me a ticket. But I am so short of cash at the moment I can't even come up with spending money. Besides, I liked working here the last time. The owner of the place, Dominique, is a woman I admire greatly. She is tough and smart. You have to agree to a long list of rules to work here (beginning, quite sensibly, with no drugs and no hooking, as both are against the law in New York), but in exchange there is a lot of creative freedom. And you can come and go pretty much as you please.

I am genuinely surprised at how much I enjoy working here. Perhaps it's the sense of balance it gives me. The kind of sex work I usually do is of the nurturing and healing variety—very *yin*. This place is about as down and dirty, in your face—*yang*—as it gets. Plus, I simply love being Alexandra. She's the archetypal opposite of Amara, my sensitive, New Age goddess persona. I also love the exercise. If I could have this much fun at a gym, I'd join one. I also enjoy hanging out in the back room with the other women, imagining that this is actually a modern temple of the sacred prostitute. I even like a lot of the clients. The ones I don't like are either bearable or ignorable, and there are always enough women working here that you can easily disappear when you want to avoid someone who's just too creepy.

So I'm looking forward to today. The entrance to the Harmony is discreet. Only a small sign above the door identifies it as a place of pleasure. I walk through the door and then through the same turnstile the paying customers must pass through. I wait for the cold blast of air-conditioning. Instead, the air is only slightly cooler than the air outside.

"What's up?" I ask the burly doorman.

"Da air conditionah," he replies in fluent Brooklynese, "is deceased."

The heat gets to me. It's very hard to maintain Grace Kelly–perfect makeup and hair in 100 degree heat and 90 percent humidity. Especially while you're dancing on someone's lap and he's even sweatier than you are. Thank goddess it's dark in here. After about four hours, I abandon any hope of maintaining the look. I retire to the back room and wipe away all my makeup except what little is left of my mascara. I put on some fresh lipstick and pull back my damp hair into what I hope might pass in the darkness for a chic chignon. I wipe the sweat off my body with a damp paper towel and head back to the floor.

I see the Cowboy even before he actually passes through the turnstile at the entrance to the club. He stands out like a cool Montana breeze against all the sweat-soaked business shirts and briefcases. The Cowboy is cute. He looks authentic. He's wearing faded jeans; scuffed, pointy Western boots; a pale, lightweight plaid shirt; and, of course, a well-worn cowboy hat. He reminds me of an older, more weathered version of Jon Voight in *Midnight Cowboy*. I am intrigued. I move in. He spots me only a few moments after I see him.

"Hi," I say.

"Hi."

"Would you like a dance?"

We find a chair. He sits. I sit on his lap. Well, not sit, actually. Half my weight is on my feet. If you actually sit on a client's lap, you can't move as well. (Then there's my ego—I wouldn't want him to think I'm *that* heavy.)

I start the dance the way I start every dance. I take a deep breath and I gaze into his eyes, specifically his left eye. I learned this technique in Tantra. A person's nondominant eye (the left eye if the person is right-handed, the right eye if they are left-handed) is considered the gateway to the soul. You don't have to worry about accidentally glimpsing their soul without their permission or allowing them unintentional access to yours. That gateway stays pretty firmly shut unless you really want to open it up. Besides, most people can't take too much eye gazing. It's just too intimate. I use it for a couple of reasons. First, it gives me a point of focus. (As a dancer and performer, you always do better work when you have a focus.) Second, eye gazing, even if it isn't returned or doesn't last more than a couple of moments, keeps me compassionate. When I look into someone's eye, I see them as so much more than a tip machine. I see their vulnerability, their hunger, their humanness. It makes the dance more of a healing experience, for me at least.

The Cowboy seems experienced at this lap dance ritual and at the same time a bit shy. He isn't hesitant, but he lacks the bravado I'm accustomed to from the Wall Street regulars. I smile. He smiles back. My eyes find his eyes. The Cowboy catches my gaze and holds it. Tight. The stripper on the stage behind me is working to a rhythm and blues tune I particularly like, and my hips pick up the beat like a wave. My breath goes along for the ride. The Cowboy's gaze stays right with mine.

The song is almost over and we're still eye-gazing. This is great! This almost never happens. *Please, please, let this continue for another song,* I plead silently. As the song ends and the next begins, I realize that the dance will indeed go on. But where's the money? Damn. He should have offered something by now. Shit, now I'm going to have to bring it up. As I'm about to speak, I feel the unmistakable touch of currency sliding between stocking top and thigh. I have no idea where that bill came from. I never saw him get it out. Thank goddess. Let's rock and roll. And that's just what the next song is, a hard-driving Springsteen tune. The wave that we have become together transforms into a tsunami. His breath matches mine as intensely as his gaze. It feels like we're held in a transparent, egg-shaped capsule that contains all our accumulated energy and feeds it back to us. My eyes are glued to his, his to mine.

Then the hallucinations start. The features of his face begin to change. Like a scene in a science fiction movie, he appears to morph into another person—and then another.

I can tell from the look in his eyes that he's having similar hallucinations about me. I have had this happen to me numerous times in Tantric rituals, but I'm surprised that he doesn't find it more frightening—I did, the first time it happened to me. But he likes it. Now he's rocking back and forth with me so intensely that I think the chair will break. I have long since stopped worrying about holding back my weight. We're entwined as one sweaty, wet, multiarmed dragon, and that dragon can fly. We're in the club, but beyond it. We hear sounds and see stars from other dimensions. Every atom in our beings vibrates with bliss. We are part of all that we can perceive and simultaneously at the center of it all. We know everything about each other and we have known each other forever in that moment. And that moment just keeps rolling.

This simply can't be happening—not here, not in this place—but it is. I'm having an authentic Tantric, full-body orgasmic, fly-me-to-the-moon-and-see-the-goddess, erotic experience on a stranger's lap in a low-rent lap dancing parlor. The second this thought flashes across my mind, I let it go. Experience has taught me that the only thing guaranteed to end a magic carpet ride like this is a critical mind. I take a big breath and look more deeply into his eyes. Our tether to the earth is cash. At the end of each song, somehow, a folded bill finds its way into my stocking top. It doesn't dampen our enthusiasm. It doesn't fuel it. It's simply part of the ritual.

Eventually we land. Perhaps he was running low on cash. Perhaps I was running low on energy. Most likely, the twenty minutes of highly aerobic activity simply burned the erotic energy out of both of us in the triple-digit heat. We sit through one more song, with me still perched on his knees, facing him. Silently. Gently rocking. Smiling. Our eyes speak our complete and utter awe at what just happened. The music still blares around us. We do not speak. He tries to pay me one more time; I push the bill back into his hand. I stand up. So does he. I want to hug him, but it just doesn't feel right. I reach out and place my right hand on his heart and give a little squeeze. He puts his left hand over mine and squeezes back. I bow my head ever so slightly and step away. He walks slowly to the exit, steps through the turnstile, and moseys off into urban Tantric history.

I was not often in the city in August. I was usually in the woods somewhere, either facilitating or participating in a workshop. I loved my long, warm workshop days. They were filled with the kind of fun and wonder you can only appreciate after too many adult years spent longing for the simple joys of summer camp. So, my workshops were actually summer camp for adults—adults who just happened to be captivated with sex, spirituality, and healing, that is. We held workshops on every imaginable New Age subject: Tantra, Taoism, Shamanism, erotic massage, breathwork, rebirthing, herbalism, Reiki, chanting, dancing, channeling, clairvoyance, clairsentience, and clairaudience. We may have been New Age, but we weren't wimps. We were workshop warriors. There was nothing we wouldn't look at, breathe through, chant out, process, or massage. We looked at our shame, our grief, our boundaries, our wounds, and our joy. We forgave, we accepted, we hugged, we orgasmed, we loved.

We lived intensely. We were grateful to be living at all.

Years of AIDS had taken their toll on all of us. We were gay, lesbian, queer, heterosexual, bisexual, two-spirit. (We weren't yet transgendered—that wouldn't come along for another five or ten years.) We were sex workers, artists, teachers, massage therapists, nurses, writers, accountants, marketing directors, corporate vice presidents, astronomers, and herpetologists. Some of us had been sexually abused; some of us hadn't. Many of us were recovering or practicing Catholics. Most of us should have been dead by now. Some of us would be soon. What we shared was a longing to reclaim our spiritual and sexual selves from the Judeo-Christian scrap heap they had landed on when "sex equals death" became the new urban motto. Most of us had lost dozens, if not hundreds, of friends and coworkers to the AIDS epidemic. And they were still dying.

I had come to this New Age out of sheer desperation. The AIDS crisis had stripped away everything I thought I could take for granted in life: my friends, my sexual freedom, my sense of safety in the world. I needed help. I needed a space to grieve and to regain my strength. Most of all, I needed a new deity. I'd pretty much lived without one since I'd run screaming from Catholicism when I was fifteen. I needed a deity who was on my side, who loved and approved of the world my friends and I lived in. I needed a deity who was queer and weird and paradoxical and kind and funny and very, very sexual. Just like me.

This desire for deity was new for me. I'd always been interested in mysticism and sex, but I kept pretty quiet about both. When I told my mother I was no longer going to pretend to be a Catholic, she was horrified. She told me I couldn't just resign. "You've been baptized!" Through her tears of anguish she warned, "You'll go to hell!" Somewhere down deep I carried that message. If I was too mystical and too sexual, that big, angry, vengeful god I'd escaped from would spot me and there would be hell to pay. Literally.

So I downplayed both my sexuality and my spirituality for nearly twenty years. But the AIDS crisis forced me to confront both. In metaphysics, we say that no matter how bad things get, there is always something to be grateful for. I'm grateful to the AIDS crisis for Tantra.

In the course of my workshop summers, I became a Tantrika. (All that means is someone who practices Tantra.) To be precise, I didn't actually *become* a Tantrika, I simply realized I had always been one. I didn't need to convert to Tantra, and I didn't need to find a church to do it in. All I needed were open eyes, deep breaths, and a sense of adventure. I didn't need a new anthropomorphized deity at all; I simply needed a sex-positive spiritual practice. I became a Tantrika because it was both logical and practical. (I may be a Pisces, but I have Virgo rising.) Tantra took me up out of the grief and the pain and the helplessness to someplace powerful and ecstatic. Tantra made me clear and strong in the face of chaos. Tantra made me wet. Tantra cut through the crap. When I shared Tantra with others, it did the same for them. And now, after my ecstatic moment with the Cowboy, it seemed Tantra worked even in lap dancing parlors.

Although I learned Tantra in lovely, peaceful, wooded retreats, I don't live in one. I have a penchant for big, boisterous, loud, overwhelming cities. I love my periodic retreats to the beach or the woods, but I can't seem to stay away from the big city. Sadly, it's very hard to do a three-day, under-the-stars, open-air Tantric ritual with a hot tub in New York City. It just doesn't happen. So whenever I tried to create a ritual like that in New York, I would inevitably feel frustrated and stupid. There had to be a way to practice Tantra authentically, effectively, and ecstatically in environments of concrete and steel.

Before I could figure out how to practice Tantra in urban (and suburban) environs, I first had to ask, "What is the essence of Tantra?" I knew it wasn't just about being in nature. Being in the midst of quiet woods or by a roaring ocean was healing and nurturing, but it wasn't nature alone that produced the passion, creativity, and ecstatic peacefulness I had found in my workshops. Nature provided me the opportunity to slow down, breathe more deeply, drop my emotional armor, and simply be more *conscious* of the beauty in each moment of the day.

Consciousness. That was it! The difference between my ordinary urban life and my wooded Tantric retreats was *consciousness*. If I could be completely conscious and present in each moment, it wouldn't matter whether I practiced Tantra in Bali or on the Bowery. Not only would location not matter, neither would strict adherence to "traditional" Tantric practices. Anything I performed with complete consciousness would be completely alive, authentic, and transformative. It was this theory that launched my search for a new kind of Tantric practice. In the pages to come, I'm going to share with you what I found: a flexible, conscious, urban Tantric practice that you can use, enjoy, exploit, adapt, expand, fold, spindle, or mutilate, as long as it works for you and brings you joy.

Introduction

Tantra is a vast and ancient subject. One could devote one's entire life to it and still have only scratched the surface. But you do not have to devote the rest of your life to the study of Tantra in order to enjoy its pleasures and perversions. You can begin to experience the yummy stuff right away. You won't need to go out and buy a lot of expensive stuff or change your wardrobe or learn to speak Sanskrit.

Tantra is a Sanskrit word that means "loom" or "weaving." Tantra can also mean "a continuous process," "the carrying out of a ceremony," a system, a theory, a doctrine, or a section of a book. As such, the word Tantra can simply refer to a treatise on any subject at all. So you'll often see it used in the titles of books that have nothing to do with the kind of Tantra we're talking about.

Even when we use the word Tantra to refer to the spiritual practice that includes sex, we're likely to find many hundreds of texts about that alone. Many are still untranslated or even undiscovered. Many of the Tantric teachings were never committed to writing at all. They were transmitted by word of mouth—from guru to disciple, often conditionally upon the disciple's promise of compete secrecy.

No one knows exactly when Tantra began. Some scholars believe the earliest texts were written three to five thousand years ago. The form of Tantra we'll be exploring began in India in the early centuries AD when the popular religions were Hinduism and Buddhism. The numerous sects of these religions all believed that enlightenment— by which they meant release from an endless cycle of rebirths—involved the renunciation of worldly pleasures. Each sect had its own opinions on which pleasures should be the most conscientiously avoided and how best to avoid them.

Tantra was quite deliberately different. Tantra promised enlightenment in a single lifetime to those who cultivated pleasure, vision, and ecstasy instead of avoiding it. Tantra, then, was not only a spiritual pursuit but also a kind of sociopolitical revolt, aimed at least in part at breaking down India's strict caste system. Tantra in India in the early days probably resembled the social revolution in America in the 1960s: experimentation with sex and drugs; group ecstatic rituals with music, dancing, and sex; loving whomever you choose regardless of race or background; and questioning the moral, ethical, and philosophical precepts of the day.

The sex, drugs, and rock and roll analogy does not stop there. The basic Hindu Tantric rite (Maithuna ritual) for the ordinary worshiper required the presence of several couples and their guru. Drugs were often smoked or drunk. There was food: fish, meat, grains, and wine. Then came the sex. A lot of sex. These rituals could go on for days. It was common for participating couples to exchange partners or to participate with temple prostitutes. The purpose of the rituals was not to enjoy greater intimacy with a spouse, but to achieve and experience the kind of oneness with a sexual partner that might be had between an individual and the rest of creation. Hence, "weaving" the two together.

Even in the early days, there were levels of Tantric practice ranging from "Tantra lite" to "all Tantra, all the time." For those seriously committed to Tantra's stated goal of achieving bliss in a single lifetime, there were intensive ritual programs involving ecstatic meditations, the chanting of mantras, complex yogic postures, mental visions (yantras), ceremonial intercourse with highly initiated partners (*dakinis* or "vessels of divine energy"), and eventually the ability to practice divine intercourse with oneself.

Ritual sex was a physicalization of the Tantric view of the creation of the world: Shiva (the god of pure consciousness) joining in sexual love with Shakti (the goddess of pure energy) gives birth to the world. I love this image—it is the most erotic beginning-of-the-world story I have ever heard. But its implications are far greater than that. Tantra views life as an ongoing process of creation; an ongoing marriage of consciousness and energy *at every level of existence*. The very essence of Tantra is contained in a few words—an excerpt from the *Vishvasara Tantra*:

What is Here is Elsewhere.

What is not Here is Nowhere.

This is one of those statements about which volumes have been written. I think there's sufficient power in its simplicity: what is spiritual is physical. What is physical is spiritual. If consciousness exists in my mind, it exists in my body. If energy exists in my body, it exists in my mind. Thus, at the heart of Tantra is the elimination of duality. In Tantra, we don't divide good and evil, matter and spirit, or male and female into opposing camps. In fact, Tantra is the only spiritual path I know of that has always acknowledged the sexes as equally powerful, everywhere, all the time.

The Tantric belief that to feel sexual excitement is to experience a taste of divine energy was a profound and revolutionary thought. It was then and it still is today. Where Tantra came from or how exactly it was practiced is a lot less important than what Tantra has given us: the notion that sex can be sacred, and that all of life can be both included and celebrated on the path to enlightenment. Inclusiveness and celebration are key factors in Tantra's increasing popularity today. However, Tantra is still misunderstood by many people.

Ten Myths about Tantra

Let's take a look at some of the myths that surround Tantra so that we can more fully understand what Tantra is and what it is not.

MYTH #1: TANTRA IS A RELIGION. If it were, I wouldn't be doing it. You do not have to join any group, take any vow, or say any special words to practice Tantra. You do not have to swear allegiance to anyone, and nothing bad will happen if you do it "wrong" or differently from other people who practice it. (Interestingly enough, the word religion derives from Latin words meaning "a healing of the wounds of separation," or "a making whole." So if that's what you're looking for from a religion, then yes, you could certainly find that in Tantra.)

Tantra is a spiritual practice. In an effective spiritual practice, the spirituality comes to you. You open yourself up to it—you don't have to chase after it. Or, as I like to think of it, the spirituality *does* you; you don't have to do *it*.

MYTH #2: TANTRA HAS TO BE DONE BY A MAN AND A WOMAN. Oh, this is a biggie. This one has kept more queer people out of Tantra than any other myth. How did this myth start? Probably because the practice of Tantra, being the path of acceptance of everything, has always embraced opposites: good/evil, sacred/profane, higher/lower, earthly/spiritual, yin/yang, light/shadow. In embracing these opposites, Tantra is able to accept and contain "all that is," which means not only the opposite poles but everything in between the poles. In our Western society, however, most everything is regarded as either/or, and there's not much in between. Nothing is more polarized than gender. Therefore, the Western mind reasons, if Tantra unites opposites, it must require "opposite" genders. As if there were such a thing as opposite genders! Gender is not two bins into one of which everyone must be dumped. It is more like a rainbow spectrum along which everyone can find the particular shade of color that looks the best on them.

Some Tantric *asanas* (positions) and *mudras* (gestures) are designed to balance the male and female aspects of the partners in a Tantric ritual. In my experience, this can be done between any two partners. Everyone has some male/masculine/yang qualities, and everyone has some female/feminine/yin qualities. The proportions can change on a daily basis. Bringing them together and balancing them before making love is not an exercise about gender, but rather an act of inner balancing and centering that helps us open ourselves to deeper intimacy.

MYTH #3: TANTRA IS COUPLES THERAPY FOR WHITE, MIDDLE-AGED, MIDDLE-CLASS, APOLITICAL, WOO-WOO, NEW AGE WORKSHOP JUNKIES. Tantra is practiced in a wide variety of styles by a wide variety of people. Contrary to popular notion, Tantra is primarily concerned with inner mystical experiences, not relationships. In the twentieth century, Tantra was reintroduced in the West by a few brave sex, gender, spiritual, and political radicals who ventured to India in search of an active spirituality that would embrace and empower everyone in all aspects of life, including the sexual and political. The practice of Tantra was once considered a supremely revolutionary act. It can be equally revolutionary today in the face of the current cultural rise of fundamentalist sex and gender politics.

MYTH #4: TANTRA AND BDSM DO NOT MIX. Do you think Tantra and BDSM are about as opposite as you can get? Remember, Tantra is based in paradox. You can enhance your Tantric practice by borrowing not only conscious sex techniques but also sensation-producing devices from the world of BDSM (bondage/discipline, dominance/submission, sadism/masochism). Both Tantra and BDSM are erotic arts of consciousness. Both arts add intensity to life and sex. Both embrace a wide variety of powerful, consensual practices. Both Tantric and BDSM rituals are about raising erotic energy. Both practices involve conscious giving and receiving. Both encourage risks—be they physical or emotional. Both erotic arts encourage personal freedom, individuality, and imagination. (For more on Tantra and BDSM, see chapter 19.)

MYTH #5: THERE'S NO REAL FUCKING. Trust me, you'll get to fuck, whatever that might mean to you. You can fuck as much and as long as you want to. If you are a man, you may appreciate that you will be able to have multiple orgasms without ejaculating, which means you can fuck a lot longer.

But the fact is, sex is a lot more than fucking. Sexual energy exists well beyond your genitals. Tantric sex is a full-body/full-spirit experience. People who practice Tantra are less genitally focused. When your entire body is pulsing and vibrating with pleasure, you're more likely to talk about the atoms in your body dancing to the rhythm of the universe than you are to describe the experience as a great fuck.

MYTH #6: IT TAKES TOO LONG. What's with those endless rituals? Well, it does take longer to create a gourmet meal than it does to microwave a frozen dinner. But you won't have to quit your job or give up your gym membership to practice Tantra. It may mean that you have to turn off the TV. One of the payoffs of a Tantric life is that you will probably find that your priorities change toward more pleasurable and meaningful relationships and activities.

Not all Tantric experiences involve rituals—long or short. However, I will be encouraging the use of ritual in this book. Ritual has been given a really bad rap. Rituals simply focus energy. Your ritual might be simple or wildly elaborate. In Tantra, you can create both a ritual and a ritual space that suit your style—and your schedule.

MYTH #7: YOU HAVE TO STUDY FOR YEARS TO GET IT RIGHT. There is no absolutely right way to do Tantra. More importantly, Tantra is not about being right. It's about being happy.

Sometimes I think there are just two kinds of people in the world: those who want to be right and those who want to be happy. It is impossible to satisfy people who want to be right unless you give them exactly what they want, exactly the way they want it. On the other hand, it is very easy to satisfy people who want to be happy. They are flexible, open to new ideas, and they don't have a fixed idea as to the way happiness "must" be achieved. The more creative the path to happiness, the better they like it. Does this sound like you now—or the way you would like to be? If so, you'll love Tantra.

It is true that your Tantric practice will deepen the more you do it. Nevertheless, most people will feel something pleasurable and new right away. Drop your expectations. If you think that Tantra will immediately make you a sex god/dess or will instantly repair a neglected relationship, you're setting yourself up for disappointment. Similarly, if you're thinking, "This works for other people, but it won't work for me," you're defeating yourself before you begin.

MYTH #8: YOU MUST HAVE A PARTNER. You already have a partner: yourself. Solo Tantra offers endless opportunities for sexual and spiritual growth. Many Tantric techniques are meant to be practiced alone, while others intended for partners can easily be adapted for one. In a solo practice, you can proceed at your own pace and focus completely on yourself. You may feel as if you are making love to the whole universe. Your solo rituals can become as important to you and as indispensable in your life as your meditation practice or your exercise routine.

If you are single and looking for a partner, these practices can help you attract someone with whom you will truly resonate by enabling you to recognize your true feelings, needs, and desires. In Tantra, you will also learn to speak your feelings and desires safely and with love.

You do not need to be in a long-term, committed relationship to do Tantra with another person. Tantra practitioners in the original Hindu Tantric rite were probably strangers prior to the ritual. They achieved Tantric intimacy by using breath, intention, and movement. So can you. Tantra will provide you with many excellent exercises to get to know someone better and will help intimacy grow in any relationship—new or established.

MYTH #9: YOU NEED A GURU TO STUDY TANTRA SAFELY. It's easy to figure out where this myth came from. Many if not most of the early Tantric teachings were never written down. You would have to become a disciple to a guru in order to learn them. The Tantra that was written down was often couched in code. Imagine the trouble you could get into practicing it literally! A guru would have been a very necessary guide, indeed. Today, many of these teachings have been decoded and recorded by scholars, gurus, and people who have studied extensively with gurus.

Do I think you need a guru? Not unless you want one. But I do think qualified teachers are extremely valuable. I have had many good and some great Tantra teachers, none of whom I have considered a guru. I have learned something important from all of them.

MYTH #10: A BOOK LIKE THIS IS NOT ABOUT REAL TANTRA. Anyone in the Western world (and some in the East) practicing what they call Tantra today is actually practicing some form of neo-Tantra, a westernized reduction of the original. Some people's practices may appear more traditional than others. They may have a guru; they may have studied in India. They may chant Sanskrit words, play Indian music, and decorate their homes with saris. And that's fine. It's a lovely way to practice Tantra if it makes you feel blissful and juicy. But the art of living Tantrically is living authentically, consciously, and sensuously. And that can be done in an infinite variety of styles and practices, all of which can bring about prolonged states of love, connection, and bliss.

A Quick-Start Guide

There are as many ways to approach Tantra and Tantric sex as there are reason for wanting to try them. However, it is helpful to first understand a few fundamentals. In Tantra, how you do sex is more important than what sex you do. This means that you'll probably need to adjust your approach to sex and your thinking about the way sex "works." That's what the chapters in the first part of this book, "Tantra: The Basics," will do. They will write Tantra on your mind and on your heart. But you do not need to read the whole section before you can have some fun.

In the remaining chapters of *Urban Tantra*, the sex gets increasingly physical. Jump in anywhere. Try out any exercise that appeals to you. If you like a more step-by-step approach, the book is organized in a more or less linear fashion, so you can start at the beginning and proceed as though you were attending your own private Tantra workshop.

But please remember that the physical/sexual Tantric exercises are simply the ways in which you implement the Tantric principles outlined in the first section. In order to experience the depths, breadths, and heights of Tantric ecstasy, make sure you have written Tantra on your mind as well as on your body.

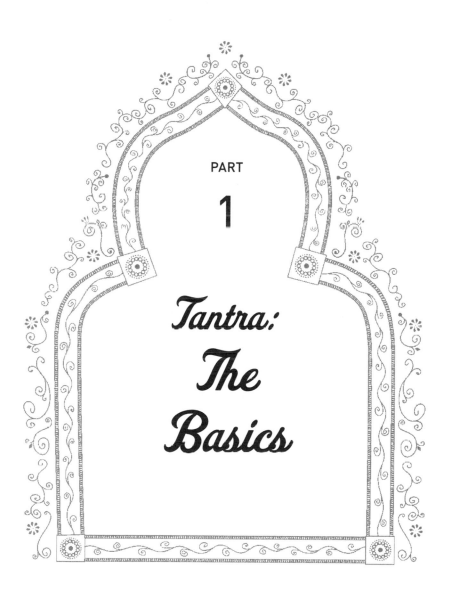

PART

1

Tantra:
The
Basics

This section of the book will tell you not only *how* to begin to practice Tantra but also *why*.

Tantra teaches us that by embracing everything in life and delving into it totally, anything can be turned into a transformative, ultimately ecstatic, experience.

We'll begin by exploring ecstasy. What is the difference between pleasure and ecstasy? Why is ecstasy important? Why might you want to prioritize the pursuit of ecstasy in your own life?

Next, I'll ask you to change your mind about how sex works. I'll introduce you to the energetic aspects of sex and give you some simple yet powerful tips on how to double your pleasure simply by changing the way you think and focus your attention.

Then I'll move to the body. You'll learn why breath, meditation, movement, and laughter are the building blocks of expanded orgasm, and you'll learn how to use them to build your own sensual stairway to paradise. You'll also learn the secrets of exquisite touch and how the way you touch can transform your relationships. Last, you'll learn how to do all of this in the time you have available in your busy schedule.

Ready? Let's get started.

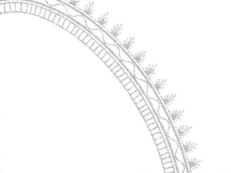

CHAPTER 1

Why Ecstasy Is Necessary

It is no surprise that one of the most popular recreational drugs is named for—and induces feelings described as—ecstasy. Humans crave ecstasy. We go to impossible lengths to achieve it, and we'll settle for almost any available substitute. This is one of the reasons sex—even bad sex—is so popular.

Ecstasy (also referred to as bliss or ecstatic bliss) is a peak experience. Peak experiences expand our possibilities. They give us permission and encouragement to reach higher and receive more. They give us a taste of our own physical power and put us in touch with our higher metaphysical power. Wilhelm Reich, in *The Function of the Orgasm*, even wrote that ecstasy in the form of total orgasm was medically necessary to the health and well-being of the human body.

Sex is not the only way to experience ecstasy, but it is certainly one of the available. Sex can give you a moment of bliss—a taste of the

GREAT

COSMIC

ORGASM.

Once you get a big enough bite of that great cosmic orgasm, you realize that sex is not the only way to have bliss. You can then find bliss in everyday, ordinary aspects of life. Osho, the visionary (and controversial) spiritual teacher, explains how sex brings us to bliss:

Because of three basic elements in sex, you come to a blissful moment. Those three are, first: timelessness. You transcend time completely. There is no time. You forget time completely; time ceases for you. Not that time ceases, it ceases for you; you are not in it. There is no past, no future. This very moment, here and now, the whole existence is concentrated. This moment becomes the only real moment . . .

Secondly: in sex, for the first time, you lose your ego, you become egoless. . . . You are not, neither is the other. You and your beloved are both lost into something else. A new reality evolves, a new unit comes into existence in which the old two are lost—completely lost . . .

And thirdly: for the first time, in sex you are natural. The unreal is lost, the facade, the face is lost; the society, the culture, the civilization is lost. You are a part of nature—as trees are, animals are, stars are. . . . You are in a greater something—the cosmos, the Tao. . . . You are just floating, you are taken by the current.

—Osho, *The Book of Secrets*

Sounds peaceful, doesn't it? It doesn't even sound like ecstasy, at least not the way we usually use the word. Ecstasy is like orgasm in that we tend to have a rather narrow definition of what the experience is "supposed" to feel like. We tend to focus on the intensely euphoric while ignoring the subtler aspects. Ecstasy is not simply the big bang of an outrageous orgasm. Ecstasy usually accompanies the afterglow of an orgasm when boundaries dissolve; when the answers to the really important questions come sailing through; when we're deeply in ourselves and aware and simultaneously outside ourselves and not ourselves. We've become part of All That Is.

Pleasure vs. Ecstasy

Pleasure, like pain, belongs to the nervous system. A sensation registers in the body as pleasant or very pleasant, painful or very painful. And sometimes, to some people, the painful is very pleasant. Whatever your interpretation, pleasure is a physical experience. The sensations of pain and pleasure are created in the body and belong to the body. Ecstasy is bodiless. It is experienced as overwhelming delight and/or inspiration. It can be a rapturous passionate feeling or a mental transport to a place of well-being, peace, or visions. It is a sense of supreme happiness felt in and by the soul. Ecstatic bliss is the joy experienced by the soul when it reconnects to Sacred Unity, to God/dess, to All That Is. Ecstatic bliss, in its purest Tantric definition, is not a feeling or a sensation. It's a metaphysical experience that occurs when all feelings, thoughts, and sensations are eclipsed by boundaryless beingness in a vast ocean of energy where everything is connected to everything else.

You can have a whole lot of extraordinary pleasure without ecstasy. It's also possible to have ecstasy without physical pleasure. But more often than not, pleasure and ecstasy have a pretty close relationship. In fact, sexual pleasure is one of the most universally available routes to ecstasy. But what makes some sex so mundane and other sex so ecstatic? Sometimes when you go into sexual pleasure totally and without any expectations, you stumble upon ecstasy. It simply happens. Is there a way to find it on a more regular basis? Yes. But before we try to find the road to ecstasy, let's look back at some of the paths on which we *haven't* found it so that we can avoid these dead ends in the future.

Adrenaline Is Not Ecstasy

Most of us live and work in a world built upon the pursuit and eventual attainment of order, logic, and success. We spend our days trying to do more in order to get more and have more. We are constantly working, studying, thinking, and planning. We have (supposedly) never been more efficient or more able to accomplish so many things simultaneously.

And we have never been more in touch. We have email, snail mail, instant messaging, telephones, faxes, mobile phones, and handheld personal computers; and new devices are being invented even as you read this. It seems we can be reached absolutely anywhere, anytime.

And yet something is missing. For all our running and grasping and striving, despite all the information instantly available to us, there's something we can't quite find, a connection we just haven't made, something we just haven't figured out yet. We know sort of what it feels like. We get a taste of it when we're right in the center of the swirling vortex of a project on deadline. We feel invincible. It's as if we have a dozen arms and three brains. We can accomplish six things at once while planning three more. We may be sleep deprived and we may not have eaten since god knows when, but that only makes us sharper. We are in the "zone"—it's all happening and it's all happening right.

We feel high and connected and powerful. That is a heck of a pleasurable buzz, but it's not ecstasy. That's adrenaline.

An adrenaline rush is that energy rush we can get when we are working hard, doing several things at once, and not eating much. It's a feeling of power, of being "on the edge," of everything being sharp and intense. Adrenaline is a hormone that also acts as a neurotransmitter, a chemical messenger used by neurons to communicate with each other and with other types of cells. It is released from your adrenal glands in relative proportion to the level of "danger" your brain perceives. Adrenaline—along with other stress hormones that accompany its release—produces arousal effects ranging from excitement to anxiety to fear, depending on the level of stimulation. The sensation you feel in an adrenaline rush is caused by the release of three chemical compounds: (1) sugar from your liver and muscles, (2) the feel-good neurotransmitter dopamine, and (3) internally created opiates called endorphins. The release of these three makes you feel alert, energetic, and euphoric. An adrenaline rush is an almost drug-like high. And unfortunately, it's just as addictive.

This stress-induced euphoria is nothing other than our prehistoric "fight-or-flight" response to extreme danger. It was meant to provide us with extra energy to get out of a life-threatening situation—it was not designed to help us make a deadline! When we live from one adrenaline rush to another, we eventually exhaust our adrenal glands and burn out. Burnout is about as far from ecstasy as you can get.

XXXtasy Is Not Ecstasy

When we see the word *ecstasy* today, it's more likely to appear on the cover of an X-rated video than in the title of a book about spirituality or healing. Not that I have anything against X-rated videos. In fact, I enjoy many genres of porn. But the thrill it provides is not true ecstasy. Neither are the highs we get from food, drugs, alcohol, shopping, X-treme sports, violent entertainment, action/adventure movies, fast cars, or thrill rides at theme parks. Obviously, in moderation, any and all of these can be simply good fun. But as a culture, we consume far too much of this faux ecstasy. Vast amounts of advertising dollars are spent on getting us to buy more and more of these cheap substitutes. Like junk food, the more we consume, the more we want. For lack of quality, we crave quantity.

So How Do We Find Real Ecstasy?

Our lives are so busy, it often seems much easier to pick up a quick ecstasy substitute than to find the time to enjoy real, gourmet ecstasy. But our beings crave real ecstasy just like our bodies crave real, nutritious food. We can only survive for so long on junk food, and on faux ecstasy, before the lack of the real thing results in illness, lethargy, and depression.

But how do we introduce real ecstasy into our already overloaded lives? The answers are simpler than you may think:

Stay in the present moment.

Don't try so hard.

Stay in the present moment.

Drop your expectations and your judgments.

Stay in the present moment.

Surrender.

Stay in the present moment.

Be more conscious.

Stay in the present moment.

Learn how to do all of this in sex . . .

. . . in the present moment.

CHAPTER 2

Be Here Now

The Buddha said that the human condition is like that of a person shot with an arrow. It is both painful and urgent. But instead of getting immediate help for our affliction, we ask for details about the bow from which the arrow was shot. We ask who made the arrow. We want to know about the appearance and the background of the person who strung the bow. We ask about many things—inconsequential things—while overlooking our immediate problem. We ask about origins and ends, but we leave this moment forgotten. We leave it forgotten even though we live in it.

We must first learn how to journey into the now.

—Steve Hagen, *Buddhism Plain and Simple*

One evening, I had dinner with three friends at the Marquis de Sade, an S/M-themed restaurant in New York City. The restaurant was a cross between a dungeon and a dining room. It had two menus: one for food and the other for play. Between food courses you could flog someone or get flogged, eat out of a dog dish or feed someone out of one, get locked into a little cage or lock someone into one, and get a spanking or give one, all under the appreciative gazes of other diners. On this particular night, an attractive leather-clad waiter was flogging a shirtless young male patron in the front room. This was a pretty common scene at de Sade, so at first I didn't pay much attention. But something about this scene captured my attention. It was so intimate that at first I thought the two participants might have been lovers. But no, this was de Sade, and waiters didn't get to flog their lovers on company time. Obviously the young man had chosen this particular erotic appetizer from the play menu.

The waiter with the whip was unwavering in his attention, dealing out each stroke with perfect intensity and waiting just long enough before giving the next. The young man was surrendering completely to the pain. He seemed to relax into the experience more with each stoke. His eyes were closed and his lips were slightly parted. His breathing would sharpen as the whip hit his back and then slow down again as the pain dispersed. The man doing the whipping (the "top") was deliberate and slow, never striking until the previous stroke had been completely absorbed. He never took his eyes off the young man, despite having to adjust his position occasionally to avoid the dinner trays speeding past him and the enthused voyeurs gathering around. It was an extraordinarily sensual and erotic performance.

Why was this scene so compelling? It wasn't particularly theatrical. It didn't "go" anywhere. Nothing dramatic happened. So why couldn't I take my eyes off it? Because it was so conscious. The top kept his attention focused on the body he was flogging, yet 10 percent of his peripheral awareness stayed in the room so that he could avoid waiters and voyeurs. He watched the young man's breath rise and fall, often matching his own to it. He watched the young man's muscles ripple and relax, which let him know when the time was right for the next stroke. He never hurried, nor did he do anything simply to entertain the crowd. He had no agenda other than to give the young man exactly the flogging he wanted. He wasn't trying to look good or get anywhere. He just gave totally. In addition, the young man was one great receiver. Having asked for what he wanted at the beginning of the scene, he went totally into the experience of receiving it. He stayed aware and present. And he breathed. He breathed a lot.

If only we could pay this kind of attention in our daily lives. But no, our minds are constantly racing like a tape player with only two speeds: fast-forward and reverse. We feel guilty about things we've done in the past and worry about all the disasters that might befall us in the future. When we are at work or school, we worry about all the things that need attention at home, and when we're at home, we worry about the work we left unfinished. Seldom do we notice anything in the present moment unless it explodes in front of us. And then we worry about when it might happen again.

It's pretty difficult to feel sexy, creative, and peaceful with all this incessant mind chatter hammering in your head. But there is good news: the same busy mind that has been making you a stressed-out mess can help you become as conscious and present in the now as the waiter and his client.

Remember: All consciousness really means is that you are in

a relaxed state of awareness with a quiet mind able to focus

gently and easily on what's going on at the present moment.

Consciousness is not some impossibly esoteric concept. It's not something granted by a guru with a touch to your third eye. It's simply the ability to focus, to put your *attention* where your *intentions* are.

Now that's easy to say, but in practice it can be pretty hard to do. How many times have you tried to focus on your lover's body only to have your mind flip away to some mundane work problem? It happens to all of us. When it comes to sex there are so many things that can distract us. First and foremost, there are fantasies. Now, I'm not saying that fantasies are bad. Fantasies are an important part of our sexual imagination. They can be extremely useful for awakening and expanding our desire. They can be used to explore new realms of intimacy and fun when you and your partner focus on making a shared fantasy come true. But if you are focusing most of your attention on the fantasy running in your head instead of on the person you are with, you are not engaged in a conscious sexual encounter.

One of my least favorite pop sex tips for men is the one about how to slow down ejaculation by thinking about something mundane or unpleasant. Talk about unconscious! Becoming more conscious of what is happening is far more effective. Conscious techniques such as slowing down, changing the way you breathe, and changing the way you thrust keep your attention focused on your pleasure and your partner. (See chapter 8 for more on delaying ejaculation.)

We want to learn to be mindful—both in sex and in life. All that means is that we want our minds to be full of the present moment and not of other thoughts. You don't have to be in a silent place completely free of distraction to be mindful. There are a few simple techniques you can use to start to be more aware, right here, right now.

Breathe

Breath is our single greatest source of energy and aliveness, yet by the time we are adults most of us are breathing just enough to stay alive. We learn at an early age that having too much energy creates problems for us. We are punished for being too loud and too active; for laughing too much and crying too hard. We learn to stifle that energy—that aliveness—by limiting our breath. The less we breathe, the less we feel. This simple numbing technique has seen us through many experiences we didn't want to be fully present for. It still does.

We all constantly regulate ourselves with our breathing, and we all do it more or less unconsciously. Our breathing automatically changes to give less fuel to any feeling that registers outside the "safe" range. This has its advantages—it protects us from reacting with acute sensitivity to every stress and strain of modern life. But it also insulates us from being sensitive to things we do want to feel. Our life becomes safe and regulated; but because we established the boundaries of this safe range when we were children, we limit our potential. As adults, we could all handle—and would probably enjoy—a whole lot more aliveness.

Our first step in learning to be more alive and in the moment is to breathe more fully. Try that right now. Take a big breath. Let it fill you from your genitals to the top of your head. Notice how you expand as you inhale. Slowly release the breath. Do you feel bigger, taller? Maybe the lights seem to get brighter. Perhaps you notice sounds or smells that weren't there before.

Now take a little teeny breath. The smallest, shallowest breath you can. You'll probably have to take more breaths in order to take in enough air. Notice how you contract when you breathe shallowly. You may find yourself hunched over, at least slightly. Perhaps you tightened your belly or shoulders or scrunched up your face. You might have felt smaller and less powerful, and perhaps you even felt a twinge of anger or sadness.

Pay attention to how you breathe.

The next time you are feeling really good,

notice how you are breathing.

The next time you are feeling angry or sad,

notice how you are breathing.

You are not at the mercy of your unconscious breathing patterns. You can change how you feel by consciously changing the way you breathe. A bit later I will introduce you to several ways of breathing that I have found to be particularly energizing, stimulating, and relaxing; but for now, just be conscious of your breathing.

Breath is vitally important when you are trying to make a connection with another person. One of the easiest ways to connect with someone else is by matching your breathing to theirs. Breath is like the rhythm of a dance. It is easier to dance with someone when you are both doing the same step. If one of you is dancing the cha-cha while the other is dancing the Balinese *legong*, you are just not going to have a connection on the dance floor.

The same thing applies to our dancing emotional bodies. When two people are breathing at the same rate, they are matching and balancing their emotional and physical states. They are agreeing to dance together, to feel together. This does not mean that they are agreeing to meld together for the rest of time, nor does it mean that they can read each other's minds (although that sometimes seems to happen). What really happens is that they begin to be able to read each other's *bodies*. In sex, touch is more easily given and more graciously received. Intuition becomes stronger. Spoken communication becomes clearer and more succinct as it becomes less relied upon. This is the beginning of two beings becoming one. Breathing with someone is not only useful in sexual situations. Any time you want to be in an empathetic relationship with someone, simply match your breathing to theirs, and you will begin to have a pretty good sense of how they are feeling.

Change Your Mind

It's often said that the most important sex organ is the brain. This is literally true, biologically speaking. Erotic energy may begin in your genitals, but it's the mind that takes over from there. The mind can say yes or no to any particular expression of erotic energy. Most of what works or doesn't work in our sex lives (and our lives in general) is based on a belief we hold in our minds. For example, as a child I was made to go to church every Sunday. The mass we went to was in Portuguese, and it never varied. Every Sunday it was exactly the same. I found it excruciatingly boring. When I became an adult, I swore I would never put myself through anything like that again. I discovered Tantra. My first teacher, Jwala, was incredibly juicy, and after the first evening I was hooked. I wanted to learn everything there was to know about Tantra. So I tried to learn all the classic asanas, mudras, and Sanskrit words. I practiced a long Tantric ritual, rigidly organized into a linear progression of politically correct poses. And I was hopelessly bored. It wasn't until I changed my mind and stepped out of the past and into the present that I could begin to experience the luscious, consciousness-altering Tantric moments I'd heard about but had been practicing too rigidly to discover.

I had to change my mind about "doing things right." I had this belief from childhood that there was only one way to practice a religion, and if I didn't do it right, I would go to hell. I was repeatedly taught that Tantra was not a religion. Rather, it was a spiritual path and a way of life. But I had only one unconscious model for anything spiritual—the Catholic Church—hardly an appropriate role model for sacred sexuality! It took time and patience and a lot of positive, calming self-talk to change my mind in the area of "doing things right." As I came to understand that my practice of Tantra was as good and right for me as anyone else's practice of Tantra was good and right for them, I was able to lighten up, loosen up, and take some risks. I stopped believing that I would land in Tantric hell if I looked a little foolish or did something "wrong."

The other thing I had to change my mind about was ritual. I had years of experiencing ritual as boring. So my early Tantra rituals were all the same: mudra after mudra, very serious and very borrring. When I finally released my belief that rituals were dull and boring, I started creating wacky, crazy Tantric events with food and toys and loud music and laughter and no Sanskrit whatsoever. Suddenly people were telling me I was throwing the best rituals in town. And just as suddenly, people were telling me I was throwing the best sex parties in town! To be perfectly honest, I have not entirely banished this old belief about boring rituals. I still take a bit of convincing when someone invites me to a ritual. And sometimes I get lazy and lapse into repeating a ritual I've done before rather than creating something new. But I have learned that there's very little more deadly to me than endless repetition. So when I'm tempted by the God of the Deadly Dull, I try to create something much more bizarre and perverted as a physical affirmation that I no longer choose to believe that rituals are supposed to be stultifying.

Do Some Affirmations

Perhaps you use them now. Perhaps they are new to you. Perhaps you think they are silly New Age hokum. If the latter is true, please change your mind about that. Affirmations are very powerful and useful.

An affirmation is a simple positive statement that you make about something that you want to create for yourself. It is stated in the present tense as though what you are affirming already exists in the present moment.

"I love myself exactly the way I am."

"Everything is working out for my highest good and for the highest good of all concerned."

"I am safe."

"My income is constantly increasing."

Every thought you think is creating your future.

If you're thinking, "I'm fat, ugly, and broke, and I'm never going to find a partner," that's what you're creating in your life. If, on the other hand, you affirm, "I am attractive, prosperous, and lovable, and I only attract loving people into my world," you will begin to create that reality. Very simple. Very powerful.

Throughout the remainder of this book, you will read example after example of affirmative language and behavior. You are completely in control of the style of language in the affirmations you wish to use. If you cannot imagine yourself saying, "I am the source of my own love," perhaps you could say, "My happiness is up to me." If "I am a beautiful and loving person" makes you gag with self-consciousness, you might say, "I totally rock! I am a love magnet!" You get the idea. The point is that we must stop beating ourselves up with what we say. How many time a day do you hear yourself or someone else say something like "I can't believe I did that. I am so stupid!" Or, when presented with the possibility of a raise or a promotion or a new lover: "Yeah, like that'll actually happen!" So next time you hear yourself say or think something negative and insulting about yourself, try to stop, forgive yourself, and create its affirmative opposite: "I am intelligent, prosperous, loving, and loved." Pretty soon you'll notice that you're treating yourself more gently and lovingly in all areas of your life.

A basic premise of Tantra is self-acceptance. Another is self-love. With these, you can create or change anything in your life. Your mind is either your most powerful ally or your worst enemy. The choice is yours.

How do you wish to use your mind?

What is it you want in your life and in your sex?

Will the thought you'll think when you look up from this page be something you want to see happen in your life?

Get clear on what you really want and start talking and acting like it already exists, because on some level it already does; it just may not have fully manifested yet. The thoughts you think today create your tomorrow—so when tomorrow comes, would you rather be greeted with your fondest dream or your worst nightmare?

However, no matter how much you love yourself or how many affirmations you say, you cannot control what others do. Sometimes things happen that make you feel powerless and sad. Whether what happened was intentional on someone's part or not, you always have the choice as to how you respond to it. If your lover leaves you, you can blame him or her for everything that's wrong in your life; or you can be grateful that their departure has created room for the person you'd be much happier with. I have found that no matter how bleak or tragic the situation, there is always something to be grateful for. For example, even though I lost nearly two hundred friends and colleagues in the AIDS crisis, I am eternally grateful for all I learned about the power of unconditional love during those difficult years. I have even heard victims of sexual abuse say that they would not be as whole, happy, and powerful today without the skills and the self-awareness they acquired in their recovery.

Here's a powerful use of affirmations worth noting: people who affirm that they are *survivors* of their sexual abuse subsequently are; they are no longer victims of it. They have not forgotten about the abuse, nor do they deny it happened. They have made a decision to no longer be victimized by it. *They have changed their minds.*

We can always change our minds, but there are situations in which we might not chose to change our behavior. A friend of mine was brutally abused by her stepfather as a child. One of his most abusive acts was to put a dog collar on her and chain her to a post in the backyard. My friend has done an astoundingly effective job of forgiving this man and transforming her life. But does she find bondage and domination play involving a leash and collar erotic? Hell no. She won't even wear necklaces. None of us is under any obligation—spiritual or otherwise—to do things we don't want to do "in order to grow as a human being." In fact, saying no can be one of the most healing things we can do, especially in sex. (It's only fair to note that I also know people who have consciously used BDSM as a powerful healing tool for their sexual abuse issues. What works for one person may not for someone else. It all comes down to making conscious choices and being willing to change one's mind.)

Focus and Imagine

By changing your mind, I mean allowing your mind to expand so that it can accept more and more possibilities—what Science of Mind teacher Eric Pace calls the "Totality of Possibilities." For example, having a breath orgasm is easy. It's believing that one is possible that can be difficult.

❋
Focused Awareness

Let's look at how we want to use our minds in the practice of Tantra. The first principle is: energy follows thought. Let me show you how this works.

1. Close your eyes.
2. Put all your attention on the little finger of your right hand.
3. Send your breath there.
4. Visualize light from one hundred stars shining into this little finger.
5. Hear the sounds inside your finger.
6. Feel the blood pulse there.
7. Do this for a couple of minutes.

How does your little finger feel? Bigger, more awake, and more alive, right? Some people describe it as feeling as if their little finger is the only finger on their hand.

Two techniques you used in that little exercise were *focused awareness* (also called *attention*) and *imagination*. The use of the two of them led to *sensation*. You *felt* a change in your little finger. I call this technique FITYFI (fake it till you feel it), and I will be encouraging you to use it many times in the course of our erotic travels. Not only can FITYFI help you create sensation, it can also help you increase sensation. Now try this little trick on your clit. Or your cock. (Or for some of you, both!)

The technique of using your mind to focus awareness and move energy through the body is incredibly powerful, and it's not limited to what you feel; it also applies to what you can do with another person. I tried a little experiment once while I was making love. (My lovers have come to accept that my research persona as a lover is both a blessing and a curse.) My lover was lying on her back. I was leaning over between her legs, tonguing her clit. She was enjoying it. I was busy writing the letters of the alphabet on her clit with my tongue (a little trick I picked up from the late comedian Sam Kinison—I owe ya, Sam). I began to visualize sexual energy traveling up her spine, over her head, down the front of her body to her clit, and up her back and around again. I was wrapping her in a kind of erotic egg of energy. She reacted almost instantly! Suddenly she began to moan and writhe, and just as suddenly, she was about to come. I had very deliberating not changed anything I was doing with my tongue and my hands had never moved.

What would happen if I stopped the visualization? I wondered. Again, I did not change anything I was doing to her clit nor did I move my hands. But I stopped visualizing the circuit of energy I had been wrapping around her. Her energy fell like a stone. I resumed my energy circle. Zoom—back to moaning and writhing. I stopped again; her energy fell. The experiment over, I tongued, "Y-o-u c-a-n c-o-m-e n-o-w," on her clit, and she did.

Make No Judgments, Make No Comparisons, and Delete Your Need to Understand

In both sex and life, I have frequently put myself in situations that have seemed crazy, weird, stupid, impossible, ridiculous, and even dangerous by the standards I grew up with. Had I listened to old judgments, I would never have experienced a breath orgasm, never made love with the fairies in the woods, never made a sexually explicit film, never fist-fucked anyone, never licked whipped cream off a roomful of women . . . well, you get the idea. I would have missed a lot.

What's more, it's all too easy to compare ourselves and our experiences to others. When I first went to an ecstasy breathing circle, I felt hopelessly inadequate. Everyone was breathing rhythmically and dancing around like children playing a game familiar to everyone but me. I didn't know the breath, the dance, or what I was supposed to feel. I felt clumsy, ignorant, and inadequate. Everyone seemed to know what they were doing, and everyone seemed to be having a better time than I was. The facilitator of the circle sensed my unease. Who knows—maybe he'd matched his breath to mine. He took my hand, and he breathed with me and danced with me for a couple of minutes.

"That's it, you're doing great. This is your first time, isn't it?" he said. "Don't try to do what anyone else is doing. Just enjoy yourself. Be in your own experience. That's the only goal."

I felt like I'd been released from a cage. Suddenly I was free. I danced any old way I wanted and breathed any old way I wanted and got bigger and wilder and happier—and by the end of the evening, I felt ecstatic indeed. Plus, I wound up making several new friends who were attracted to my sense of abandon and silliness.

It's easy to avoid trying something new because you don't understand how it works or how it *could* work. Many seemingly impossible things happen when we start raising sexual energy. Peoples' faces appear to change. We see, hear, smell, and feel things that may or may not "really" be there. We have sudden bursts of emotion or sensation that appear to have no cause or connection to the feeling preceding it or following it. Sometimes we see the Divine. It's so unlike our everyday reality, it's like we've entered a parallel universe. Furthermore, who would have ever thought that getting blindfolded or tied up or whipped could produce deeply satisfying feelings of peace and contentment? Or that some breathing and a few yoga-like positions could make you feel like you'd been blasted to another galaxy? It's easy to be skeptical. Easy, but not smart. Nothing great has ever been achieved by affirming, "That's ridiculous; it won't work." Lots of things are ridiculous and many of them work. So try something ridiculous. What's the worst that can happen? You might look foolish? Get used to it. We all wind up looking foolish once in a while, especially during sex. As my dear friend and frequent teaching partner, Chester Mainard, says, "Blushing is good for the complexion. It brings all that nice blood up into the face to nourish the skin." So start signing up for some foolishness facials and watch your bliss level rise.

Repeat often: I make no judgments, I make no

comparisons, and I delete my need to understand.

Drop Your Expectations

When we think we know what is going to happen or that we can make something happen, we set ourselves up for disappointment. Despite the cultural proclivity for multitasking, the mind can actually only focus on one thing at a time. You miss what *is* happening in the present moment if your mind is busy writing a script for how things *should* turn out.

Allow me to illustrate. My friend Chester was facilitating an erotic massage workshop. A group of two dozen or so erotic explorers had spent the weekend learning and practicing erotic massage, ecstasy breathing, and an amazing Taoist breath orgasm technique called the Clench and Hold. Over the course of the three-day workshop, everyone had been both giver and receiver in a ritual that combined all three techniques. One participant had had a particularly wonderful time receiving. She had finished each ritual with a Clench and Hold and had gone into intensely pleasurable orgasmic states, each one more amazing than the one before. Now the weekend was almost over; there was just one more chance to receive. As she got on the massage table, she prepared herself for the orgasm of her dreams, the blast-off of all blast-offs, her ticket to a private audience with the goddess: the ultimate cosmic orgasm.

The massage progressed nicely. She asked for what she wanted and received an enthusiastic erotic massage. She took big, full breaths and used every technique she had ever learned to move sexual energy. Then she finished up with a huge Clench and Hold and waited for her reward. And waited. Nothing happened. She waited some more, searching for her cosmic orgasm. Still nothing. Behind closed eyes she kept trying, but nothing happened. No big experience. Finally, thoroughly disappointed, she gave up. When she got off the table she reported to Chester what had happened. She had seen nothing, heard nothing, felt nothing, thought nothing. It was as though she didn't even exist. Literally nothing happened.

"And that was bad?" asked Chester.

"No, not bad, exactly," she replied. "After I gave up, it was actually peaceful. But it was so disappointing."

"Let me understand," said Chester. "You felt egoless, you experienced no-mind, and you found inner peace. That was disappointing? Good goddess, girl, what were you looking for?"

Remember: Life rarely turns out the way

we planned. Why should sex?

Release your expectations.

Giving and Receiving

Think of a deeply satisfying sexual experience you have had—something that expanded your idea of how much pleasure you were capable of. Which moment in that experience do you remember as exceptional? That moment might have lasted just a few seconds, or much longer. Focus on that moment.

I'll bet that this moment happened when you were doing nothing but receiving. You were not trying to give back to the person who was giving to you. You were not planning what you were going to do later to please your lover. You were totally and completely receiving every drop of pleasure you were being offered.

This is a good example of our inability to give our full attention to two things at once. You cannot focus on receiving if you are trying to give. Nor can you go totally into giving to your partner if you are trying to receive at the same time. In the totality of your receiving, you may give your partner a lot of pleasure. In the process of giving, you may get a lot of pleasure. But sex is a lot more satisfying when your *intention*—either to give or to receive—is clear.

Some readers might say, "But I thought the whole point of sex was to give and receive pleasure simultaneously." Well, think about it. How successful has that been for you? I know for me, the messiest, least satisfying sexual situations have been when I was trying to give to my partner who was simultaneously trying to give to me. When I was trying really hard to give, I felt that I wasn't a very good lover if I couldn't get my partner to lie back and enjoy what I was offering. Then when I was trying really hard to receive, I felt guilty—guilty about taking too long to come, guilty about receiving more than I was giving—guilty about receiving too much pleasure.

After facilitating more Erotic Awakening workshops than I can easily count, I think I can safely and surely say that most people find it much easier to give than to receive. The popular belief used to be that women were especially prone to overgiving and underreceiving. While there is a lot of truth in that, I don't think men are all that far behind. Most of us seem to carry some sort of automatic guilt alarm that goes off when we are receiving pleasure. The irony of this is that the vast majority of people love giving to a receptive, willing partner who's truly enjoying her or himself. So in trying to give back while someone is trying to give to us, we are actually depriving our partner of the pleasure of being able to go totally into the experience of giving. Aren't we silly?

In coming chapters, we'll practice how to go totally into giving and then totally into receiving. Then we'll practice giving and receiving alternately in shorter intervals. But before we practice, we need to grasp the concepts of *conscious* receiving and *conscious* giving.

Receiving is not a passive activity. Receiving is not lying back, tuning out, disassociating, and letting someone do whatever they want to you. Conscious receiving is about staying awake and completely present in the moment, asking for what you want, and giving your partner feedback along the way.

Asking for what you want is not a demand or an ultimatum. It's a

sincere request that your partner may honor or politely decline.

Similarly, giving is not about forcing someone to accept things that you want to do, your way, without their enthusiastic consent or agreement. Giving is about asking your partner what she or he would like to receive, and then agreeing on what you are or are not willing to give. Giving is staying present and asking for feedback, such as "Would you like that a little harder?" or "Is that too ticklish for you?"

When you're receiving, go totally into receiving. Receive it all.

When you're giving, go totally into giving. Give everything.

In Tantra, we often speak of surrender. Surrender, even to the Divine, is something our culture does not encourage. Surrendering to the Divine means crossing over from our well-defined roles and worlds into the realm of the gods, where everything is possible and nothing is explained. Scary stuff for many of us. The word *surrender* has been commandeered by the military and the government; it conjures up images of defeat rather than release. In Tantra, surrender doesn't mean voluntarily submitting to unpleasant experiences. Surrender is not at all the same as "grin and bear it." Surrender is a conscious choice.

Some people find it much easier to surrender when that surrender is explicit, such as in S/M and bondage. Other people find that kind of explicit surrender brings up all their control issues. Everyone's path to surrender is different. Do not judge yourself for your preferences. You don't have to do things that feel wrong in order to "grow." As you develop your particular Tantric path, you may feel drawn to try new things. Great. You may also decide you never want to try some other things. Also great. That's conscious giving and receiving. That's conscious sex.

There is no goal in Tantra. Although Tantric positions, exercises, and rituals may give you bigger, longer orgasms, more intimacy with your partner, and even enlightenment, none of these are goals. While there is no goal, there is a likely outcome of Tantric practice: the kind of freedom that exists only in the present moment. You need only be present in each moment and notice what is going on. That's all.

CHAPTER 3

Know Thy Chakras, Know Thyself

We human beings have always been fascinated with our bodies and how they work. We have developed countless theories and systems to explain every observable process from birth to death. Some people believe that the chi that flows through our energy meridians is the essential life force. Others think that it's the blood flowing through our veins or the neural transmitters that send instant messages along our nerves. Tantrikas believe that our life-force energy is the Kundalini spiraling up our chakras. In Tantra, we view the body in energetic as well as physical terms. The mind, body, and spirit are all connected and engaged in every aspect of our lives, including sex.

The Seven Chakras

In Sanskrit, the word *chakra* simply means wheel. Chakras are seen—by people who can see such things—as spinning spirals of energy in the etheric body (which is located outside the physical body, about six inches to the front and back), approximately in the same areas as the glands of our endocrine system. There are seven major chakras and forty-three less significant ones. Each has numerous specific properties, including color, sound, and vibrational speed. Additionally, each chakra is linked to a specific area of the body and the emotional issues contained there. We are going to look at the seven major chakras and their primary qualities.

The first three chakras—the lower chakra—are concerned mostly with the physical world. They vibrate at slow speeds and their associated sounds are low in pitch. The higher chakras—five through seven—are more connected to the nonphysical world. These chakras vibrate at faster speeds and their sounds vibrate at increasingly higher pitches. The fourth chakra is the bridge between the two worlds.

The chakra system is a simple, practical way to direct energy and awareness to specific areas of your body. If you want to be able to move erotic energy throughout your body in order to experience a full-body orgasm, you'll need to open up the energy pathways that will make that possible. Working with the qualities of each chakra will help you do that. The properties of the chakras are also useful diagnostic tools. When I was first experimenting with one particular ecstatic breath technique, I would get a terrible headache between my eyes every time I approached orgasm. This area of the body is the third eye or sixth chakra, the chakra of intuition. Knowing this, I realized I was overusing my mind and undervaluing my intuition, not only in sex but in other areas of my life. I also realized that the breath I was using was too powerful. I was trying to force open a chakra that needed a more gentle awakening. By approaching the chakra from both the physical and metaphysical angles, the headaches soon stopped, my intuition strengthened, and I was able to move energy up through my third eye.

THE FIRST CHAKRA

The first chakra is known in Sanskrit as Muladhara. (Okay, I know I said I wasn't going to ask you to learn Sanskrit, but if you decide to learn more about traditional Tantra and/or the chakras, you'll find it really helpful to know the Sanskrit names.) It is located on the perineum between the anus and the genitals.

Color: red
Sound: low in pitch; C on the Western musical scale
Physical focal points: base of the spine, legs, feet, rectum,
   and immune system
Metaphysical aspects: grounding and survival

The first chakra is concerned with security and survival—the basic elements of life. On a personal level, the first chakra reflects issues of home, survival, and safety. On the community level, it is the "tribal" chakra, concerned with issues of family, school, job, religion, nationality, politics, and patriotism. The first chakra is also concerned with money issues, insofar as money is connected to our survival, our safety, and our tribe(s).

The first chakra grounds us like the roots of a tree: the stronger and deeper its roots, the more blossoms above. It also functions as our internal seismograph, and through it we can pick up global stresses such as revolutions, environmental disorders, terrorist attacks, and plane crashes.

Weaknesses in this chakra will manifest physically in the lower back (sciatica, for example); in problems with the hips, legs (including varicose veins), knees, and feet;

and as colon cancer and immune system disorders. In addition to physical problems, there are emotional consequences when a chakra is stressed. In the first chakra, these are related to home and belonging. You may not feel safe at home or you may have a fear of being homeless. You may fear that you will lose your job; therefore your income; therefore your home. You may feel overly possessive of your lover, believing that if your lover leaves, you will die. Or you may have trouble making your ideas take physical form. Any of these may result in depression.

Some things you can do to nourish this center are

* Standing barefoot and having someone else stand on your feet
* Seeing your spine as a column of light rooting you to the center of the earth
* Learning and practicing tai chi or bioenergetics
* G-spot massage
* Prostate massage

Here are some affirmations to strengthen this chakra:

* I let life provide everything I need.
* I always have the perfect home and I am perfectly at home wherever I am.
* I am safe.

THE SECOND CHAKRA

Known as Svadhistana, the second chakra is located at the lower abdomen, just below the navel.

Color: orange
Sound: low in pitch, one step higher than the first chakra; D on the Western musical scale
Physical focal points: pelvis, ovaries and uterus, testes and prostate, lower intestine, and bladder
Metaphysical aspects: sexuality, relationships, creativity, and power

Although this is most commonly referred to as the sex center, issues of power and control also dominate this chakra, specifically power and control over the outside world. The most creative of the lower three chakras, this is the chakra that provides the impetus from which you conceive not only a child but also the plans, desires, and dreams for all aspects of your life (which become more fully realized in the fifth chakra, the chakra of creative expression). Challenges to this chakra include rape, incest, and events energetically similar to those. For instance, not everyone has been raped, but everyone has experienced having their boundaries violated or felt a lack of privacy. It's simply a matter of degree. Constant criticism of a person's creative endeavors, accomplishments, or physical appearance is also a form of energetic rape or incest. People who grow up hearing that they will never amount to anything often suffer impotence, reproductive problems, and financial difficulties later in life.

Money is also a factor in the second chakra, but here the money issues are about relationships and power. Lower back pain—a first chakra issue because of its connection to security—is also a symptom of a financial imbalance in relationships, so it appears in this chakra as well as the first. Sex and money are also closely related. Have you ever noticed that many people feel more sexual when they make money and less sexual when they lose it? Making money makes most of us feel powerful; losing it makes us feel out of control.

Sexual shame is also a power issue. Our shame and embarrassment about sex comes from voices of authority scattered throughout our past. The sources are endless: parents, school, church, the legal system, and so on. All these authorities exert considerable control over us, or they have at one time. They were not to be disobeyed without serious consequence. The fear of being caught masturbating or reading some porn—even the fear of being caught doing *anything* sexual—can unconsciously persist throughout our lives and raise havoc with the natural expression of our sexual energy and desire.

Speaking of power, this is also the chakra concerned with the military. Not surprisingly, it's also the chakra where people usually wear their guns.

Other physical problems in the second chakra include prostate cancer, impotence, ovarian and uterine cancer, vaginal problems, and urinary problems.

Some things you can do to nourish this center are

* Talking about sex with the intention of releasing shame
* Deep-tissue massage
* Belly dancing
* Exhilaration Meditation and Cathartic Meditation (see chapter 4)
* Reichian therapy

Here are some affirmations to strengthen this chakra:

* I rejoice in my divine sexuality.
* My income is constantly increasing.
* I only attract loving, positive, sensual people into my life.

THE THIRD CHAKRA

Also known as Manipura, the third chakra is located at the solar plexus.

Color: yellow
Sound: medium-low in pitch; E on the Western musical scale
Physical focal points: stomach, pancreas, adrenals, gall bladder, liver, and upper intestines
Metaphysical aspects: self-esteem, courage, and trust

The third chakra is associated with self-respect, self-confidence, and emotions. Fear and anger are the emotions we are most likely to hold in this chakra. When this chakra is healthy and balanced, we feel safe to express our emotions without dumping them onto others. We feel brave, but we do not bully people. We have the courage to face both our inner and outer worlds. We are able to both see and deal with issues beneath the emotions we feel.

As children, the adults around us modeled the expression of emotion. Did your parents or caretakers stuff their emotions? Did they scream about every little thing? Was there a lot of fear in your house, or were your parents self-assured and confident? How were you treated when you expressed your emotions? Were you told to shut up? Were you ignored? Whether you tend to be overly emotional today, or whether you tend to run from big expressions of emotion, you can use the knowledge of your past to gain insight about how and why you deal with emotion the way you do today. And then you will be able to change your behavior if you want to.

The third chakra is also the lower chakra of intuition. It's not where we pick up the higher intuitive whisperings of our soul (that's handled in the sixth chakra), but rather those gut feelings that tell us how to move through the physical world safely. This is also the chakra of self-esteem. When we feel strong, self-confident, and brave, we respect ourselves and listen to our "gut feelings." We trust the process of life. When we aren't feeling so good about ourselves, we tend to equate who we are with the amount of power we feel we *don't* have. When we don't trust that we are strong enough or good enough to get what we want, we resort to manipulating behavior as defense. We may settle for less than we deserve in sexual relationships. We may feel afraid of the strong emotions that accompany sex.

The physical problems that manifest in this chakra are ulcers and other stomach and digestive disorders. Things "eat away" at you and you "can't stomach" things. You have a "bad feeling in the pit of your stomach" when you contemplate change.

Some things you can do to nourish this center are

* Feeling the fear and doing it anyway
* Pounding a pillow
* Screaming underwater
* Laughing
* Rebirthing (a conscious breathing process designed to release stored stress, pain, and emotional trauma)

Here are some affirmations to strengthen this chakra:

* I trust my inner voice. I am strong, wise, and powerful.
* It is safe to express my emotions.
* I am brave, I am brave, I am brave.

THE FOURTH CHAKRA

The fourth chakra, or Anahata, is located at the center of the chest, above the breast. It is also known as the heart chakra.

Color: green
Sound: mid-range in pitch; F on the Western musical scale
Physical focal points: chest, thymus, heart, lungs, breasts, arms, and hands
Metaphysical aspects: compassion and love

This is the chakra of the heart, of forgiveness, and of compassion. It's associated with following your heart, creating your heart's desire, and coming from the heart. The fourth chakra sits right in the middle of the chakras—there are three above it and three below. It is the bridge between the physical and nonphysical worlds.

In this chakra, we move beyond ourselves—beyond even our tribe. We include others; we see the bigger picture. When this chakra is in balance, we care both about and for other people, but we do not sacrifice our own health and well-being to take care of others. We feel loving and connected to others, not used by them. We may feel hurt, abandoned, or betrayed, but we are able to find acceptance and forgiveness. Sexually, we feel balanced—we give and receive with equal ease.

The emotional challenges of the heart chakra are resentment, guilt, and grief. We spend our lives learning to love. Some of the lessons are more challenging than others. When we haven't yet mastered a lesson in love, we either resent the person assigned to teach us the lesson, or feel guilty and/or sad because we can't fill all the needs of someone we love. We usually interpret the latter as meaning we don't love enough.

Heart problems—especially heart attacks—are physical challenges of the fourth chakra. Congestive heart failure is a physical manifestation of self-blame, guilt involving failures, and unexpressed sad emotions. Heart attacks are frequently the result of the type of mental/emotional conflict that can arise from a belief such as "compassionate people can't make a profit." Not surprisingly, heart problems have traditionally been the biggest killer of men, although women are catching up now that they are in the workplace dealing with the same pressures as men.

Breast cancer is another challenge in this chakra, all too common among women who feel guilty that they can never do enough for other people, while at the same time denying their own needs.

Lung problems including cancer, asthma, and pneumonia are often the result of unresolved grief.

Some things you can do to nourish this center are

* Selfloving, with a focus on bringing sexual energy up to the heart
* Yoga practices that focus on the breath
* Rebirthing
* Crying

Here are some affirmations to strengthen this chakra:

* Compassion and wise love fill all the rooms of my heart.
* I bless all of my life with love.
* I am enough, I do enough, I have enough.
* The heart cannot be broken; only barriers around the heart can be broken.

THE FIFTH CHAKRA

Also known as Vishuddha, the fifth chakra is located at the throat.

Color: blue
Sound: mid-to-high in pitch; G on the Western musical scale
Physical focal points: throat, thyroid, mouth, gums, and teeth
Metaphysical aspects: communication, creativity, and choice

The fifth chakra is the creative chakra of the upper four chakras. It is the center of our creative expression, of the spoken word, of action, and of choices and will. Every decision we make is a creative choice and has a consequence. Our decisions create our lives either beautifully or badly. This chakra sits between the head and the heart. When our head and our heart are working in harmony, we express ourselves clearly and lovingly and make decisions that help our highest dreams come true. When out of balance, we become judgmental, critical, and ill. Have you noticed how many illnesses begin with a sore throat? Perhaps the ultimate imbalance of this chakra of choices and will is addiction. It is no surprise that addictions are so prevalent in society right now. Our entire culture seems caught in a tug-of-war between the loving thing to do (heart) and the practical thing to do (mind). This conflict trickles down to each of us in countless ways every day.

Whatever decision you made a moment ago, you can make a new one right now. It's important to remember that the point of power is always in the present moment. We are always able to change. What we need is the willingness to change and the faith in the decisions we make.

As this is the chakra of creative expression, we can feel deeply wounded when we are criticized for our originality and inventiveness, or for simply speaking our truth. This is especially true in sexual situations, in which the heightened level of physical arousal makes us particularly sensitive to criticism.

This chakra is also known as the "third ear" or the "voice that listens." You know the kind of speaker who seems to be able to put into words what you know and feel but haven't been able to express? That's a speaker with a voice that listens. When our fifth chakra is open and clear, we can all express ourselves with our third ear.

The physical problems most often seen in this chakra are sore throat, gum and teeth problems, TMJ (temporomandibular joint) syndrome (commonly known as grinding your teeth), laryngitis, swollen glands, and thyroid problems.

Some things you can do to nourish this center are

* Practicing asking for what you want in sexual situations
* Drumming
* Singing and chanting
* Engaging in playful creativity
* Meditation

Here are some affirmations to strengthen this chakra:

* I express my creativity.
* I express myself easily and joyously.
* I make decisions easily and I follow through with love.
* I am willing to change.

THE SIXTH CHAKRA

Also known as Ajna, the sixth chakra is located at the forehead, between the eyebrows. This chakra is also called the "third eye."

Color: purple
Sound: high in pitch; A on the Western musical scale
Physical focal points: brain, pineal gland, eyes, ears, and nose
Metaphysical aspects: intuition and wisdom

The sixth chakra reveals your highest intuitions, insights, and visions. By nourishing your third eye, you can hear the calling of your soul. Through this eye, you can "see" just who you are. You can "see" the nature of your true calling. As such, it is the sixth chakra that nourishes your uniqueness, your divine independence, and your ecstatic nature.

This chakra is nourished when you are encouraged and permitted to follow your intuition. When the sixth chakra is out of balance, the mind tries to take over the job of the psychic center, and logic overcomes your intuitive voice. This is not to say we want to disregard the mind or make it less important than our intuition. The challenge and secret to this chakra is the integration of conscious and unconscious insights. When the two are in balance, we are capable of real creative thought; we are truly "open-minded." This is wisdom.

Our ears and eyes provide us with raw information about the world and the people around us. When the sixth chakra is clear, we are able to process that raw information with emotional intelligence so that we can learn from our experiences. We are able to evaluate our own insights, and we are open to the ideas of others. We perceive the difference between truth and illusion.

This is also the chakra of visions. Bringing sexual energy up to the sixth chakra can produce intense insights into inner and outer worlds, as well as strengthen your faith in your intuition and your personal visions for your future.

The physical challenges of this chakra are strokes, brain tumors, blindness, deafness, learning disabilities, and seizures, as well as less catastrophic headaches and sight problems. Incidentally, the pineal gland craves light. A tiny endocrine gland located in the brain, the pineal gland produces and secretes melatonin, which regulates the body's internal physiologic clock, including the sleep/wake cycle. So make sure to get enough sunlight, especially in the winter.

Some things you can do to nourish this center are

* Practicing sex magic (see chapter 22)
* Sleeping outdoors
* Getting lots of sunlight
* Practicing witnessing (see chapter 4)

Here are some affirmations to strengthen this chakra:

* I am divinely guided in everything I do.
* I let my inner wisdom guide me.
* I see and hear the love and joy around me.
* I see everything I need to see.

THE SEVENTH CHAKRA

Also known as Sahasrara, the seventh chakra is located at the top of the head. It is also called the "crown" chakra.

Color: white
Sound: very high in pitch; B on the Western musical scale
Physical focal points: pituitary gland
Metaphysical aspects: bliss, higher love, and spirituality

It is said that our spirit enters the physical body through the crown chakra at the moment we are born and leaves through the same portal when we die. The seventh chakra is the chakra of the ultimate orgasm: death by complete surrender; death and ultimate bliss. Death in this sense is usually a symbolic death—often a death to the feelings of separation, releasing you to the next level of spiritual maturity. Opening the crown chakra does not necessarily mean that your physical body will die. The seventh chakra is the door to the Collective Unconscious, and when it is open, it is your connection with All That Is. Have you ever heard someone describe their experience of an orgasm as being shot out the top of their head into a peaceful place where they felt completely at one with the universe? That is a crown chakra opening. Our death-negative culture has produced a bliss-starved population. In order to have a strong, open crown chakra, we need to regard death as powerfully and positively as we regard birth.

You don't have to believe in any particular kind of deity in order to have a strong crown chakra. Your source of inner guidance can come from a trust in some greater presence, system, or flow. Whatever provides you with a faith that

* Ultimately, everything will be okay
* Everything is unfolding exactly as it is supposed to
* You are part of something greater

will nourish the crown chakra as the precious and tenuous connection between the physical and the spiritual.

The disorders connected with the crown chakra are more energetic than physical. When they do manifest physically, they tend to be mysterious and hard to diagnose, such as chronic exhaustion; listlessness and disinterest in life; and extreme sensitivity to sound, light, or other environmental factors. Spiritual crises are more common, including the proverbial "dark night of the soul."

Some things you can do to nourish this center are

* Orgasm
* Practicing dying and pretending to be dead
* Anointing your crown chakra with essential oil of rose, sandalwood, or patchouli
* Meditating

Here are some affirmations to strengthen this chakra:

* I feel my connection to the infinite.
* I am one with the universe and all of life.
* I surrender to the process of life.

Sex and the Chakras

Sex is as much or more of an energetic event as it is a physical experience. As such, Tantra places as much focus on the chakras as it does on the physical body. However, you do not need to wait until all your chakras are perfectly clear and balanced to experience the pleasure of sexual energy rising up and flowing throughout your body. As you begin to practice the breath and energy-building exercises in the next chapter, you may notice that some chakras seem more "stuck" or "blocked" than others. Do not overanalyze the blockages. Simply focus on your pleasure and on building sexual energy. Later you can meditate on any possible connections between these weaker or blocked chakras and your emotional life, any physical illnesses you may be experiencing, and/or your personal and professional relationships.

As you begin to practice Tantra, you will notice that the practice itself helps you to heal and balance your chakras. As your chakras open up and begin spinning optimally, you'll see not only how much more mind-blowing sex can be, but how much more exciting and fulfilling all aspects of your life can be when your orgasmic energy flows freely through your body, mind, and spirit.

It's now time to explore some simple techniques that are guaranteed to kick-start the awakening and enlivening of your body, mind, and spirit.

CHAPTER 4

Wake Up Your Body, Calm Your Mind, and Free Your Spirit

In this chapter, we'll look at three of the easiest and most powerful paths to pleasure: breath, meditation, and silliness. To the Western mind, these might sound like the unsexiest erotic techniques ever proposed, but trust me, the power you will find in them is unmatched by any vibrator or other sex toy or even your hottest dream-come-true lover.

The Basics of Breath

Breath is powerful. It can produce so much extraordinary pleasure that it will amaze you. Once you become familiar with moving erotic energy around on your breath, you'll find all your erotic encounters to be much more fulfilling. Your orgasms will be longer and deeper. Eventually, you'll find yourself using breath techniques in nonerotic situations to bring erotic energy to more and more areas of your life.

❋

A New Way to Breathe

Let me give you an example of how changing the way you breathe can change the way you feel.

1. Sit comfortably. You're going to yawn. A yawn is your body's way of asking for more air. More air means more aliveness. The next time someone yawns while you're talking,

don't be offended; thank them. It means that they're trying to be more present and alive for what you are saying.

2. Yawn. Try it. Let a really big yawn happen to you. Fake it until you feel it, but do not force it. Come as close as you can to a really big yawn.

3. Feel how the yawn opens the back of your throat and stretches out your whole mouth and face. That's the feeling of openness you want.

4. Now breathe. Let your mouth fall open slightly. Relax your jaw and face, open the back of your throat, and breathe in through your mouth, gently but fully.

5. Exhale. Don't push the breath out; just let it fall out with a gentle little sigh: *ahh*.

6. Take in a much air as you can, as effortlessly as you can, and then let it go.

7. Keep breathing. Continue for three minutes.

Notice how you are feeling. Do you feel any different from when you started? Are you a little dizzy now? Lightheaded? Spacey? Relaxed? Weird? Do you feel good? Or not?

If the breath made you a little lightheaded, did that worry you? There's no need for concern. Couldn't you benefit from being a little lighter in the head? I know I could.

Changing the way you breathe produces a perceptible change in consciousness. It's a physical reality. So, changing the way you breathe changes the way you feel. Sometimes it makes you feel out of control. Most of us walk around in this world trying to maintain total control over our bodies, to the extent that we have reduced our breathing to a level just deep enough to keep us going. It's not just an individual choice—it's cultural. Imagine this: you're going to work one morning and just like always, you step into the crowded elevator. The door closes. But this morning, someone in the rear of the car takes a huge, deep breath and exhales with a loud *ahh*! What would you think? What might everyone else think? Would that breath seem strange and out of place? Why? In response to a sex-negative, body-shy culture, we have reduced our breathing to a survival level. We take in just enough air to stay alive. Given today's obsession with eating and dieting, I suspect that we have replaced our need for air with a desire for food. Perhaps if we breathed more, we would eat less.

We unconsciously hold our breath many times each day. In fact, that is usually the first thing we do when we don't want to lose control of some situation. It's part of a reflex we all seem to have that causes us to tense up and "get through it." Unfortunately, it's also the technique most of us use when we "try" to have an orgasm. We bear down, hold our breath, and try to "make" ourselves come. Sure, you can have an orgasm that way. Most of us have. But deep, full, extended orgasms happen more easily and naturally as a result of the dance between tension and release, contraction and expansion.

When used consciously, both tensing up and holding your breath can lead to a mind-blowing orgasm after the body has been charged up with lots of breath. Energy pathways open, and the orgasmic energy can travel where we direct it. There's a difference between the kind of orgasm you have after a five-minute masturbation quickie under the covers when you're trying not to make any noise, and after a loud, passionate, energetic romp with a hot lover. In the former instance, the orgasm is primarily happening in and around your genitals. That's as far as the orgasmic energy can travel in a short time with minimal breath. In the latter instance, the orgasm may feel like it is happening all over your body and shooting out the top of your head. That's what happens when your energy pathways have been opened up and you have expanded to allow more energy.

The amount of breath involved is not the only reason for the difference between these two orgasms. In the second example, we also added the energy-building elements of movement, sound, and a partner. However, when we move, make sounds, and relate with another person, we also breathe more, exponentially increasing the energizing effects.

Changing the way you breathe will sometimes produce an extreme change of consciousness, so it pays to discover which kinds of breathing will produce which kinds of changes of consciousness. Some breath techniques will calm you down; others will energize you. For example, mouth breathing is a charging mechanism. We breathe through the mouth when we need or want more oxygen—for pleasure as well as survival. Although it is considered linked to our response to stress, breathing through our mouths involves more than the primitive human fight-or-flight response. Have you ever seen people in the throes of passion with their mouths closed, breathing through their noses? Of course not. Mouth breathing charges the body. When you breathe through your nose, air goes to the lower lobes of your lungs and stimulates the vagus nerve, part of the parasympathetic nervous system: the body's rest-and-restore system. The parasympathetic nervous system lowers heart rate and blood pressure, and sets in motion other calming measures to allow the body to rest, recover, and gain new energy.

Four Conscious Breaths

Following are four kinds of breath that I can count on to provide delicious, body- and consciousness-altering experiences on a regular basis.

Practice each of the following breaths for five to ten minutes at a time, with the exception of the Breath of Fire, which you should practice only for a minute or two at a time. While you practice, keep in mind these general guidelines:

* Keep your eyes open and focused gently at a point across the room so that you stay focused on your breathing and don't nod off or space out.
* Set a timer so that you don't have to keep track of the time.
* When your time is up, take three deep breaths, and then just breathe normally.
* Notice how you feel after each of the four conscious breaths.
* Breathe through your mouth while you are learning each breath (except for the Breath of Fire, which is always done through the nose). When you become familiar with the breaths, you can experiment with nose versus mouth breathing.

The Bottom Breath

Practice for five to ten minutes.

Bottom breathing is a gentle, easy way to calm you down and open up your senses. It's the ideal breath to use when you want to move out of the busy or stressful state of doing into the easy, relaxed awareness of being.

1. Sit on the floor with your legs crossed (or on a hard-backed chair with your feet flat on the floor) and your spine straight. With your hands, pull the fleshy part of your buttocks aside so that you are sitting on your sit bones. (Once you learn the breath you can do it in any position.)
2. Place your hands on your belly. Relax your belly. Just let it go. Let it be round in your hands. (Despite the culture's fascination with concave bellies, bellies are supposed to be at least slightly rounded.)
3. Begin by exhaling all the air out of your lungs.
4. Then, as you inhale, very gently push out on the anal sphincter. Imagine that your anus can "kiss" the floor or the seat of the chair.

5. On the exhale, don't do anything. Don't contract your anus; don't hold it; don't push. Do nothing. Just let go.
6. Repeat. On the inhale, push out with the anal sphincter; on the exhale, do nothing.
7. Keep going.

That's all there is to it. If you find it hard to focus on your anus, try focusing on your belly button—it's doing the same thing. As you breathe in, your belly button and your anus move outward. As you exhale, they return to their original position without any effort on your part.

This breath may take a little while to get used to, as we are not used to focusing on our anuses. Although it may seem a little odd, this is actually a very natural breath; it's just not one you usually do when you are awake. This is how you breathe when you are sleeping deeply. If you watch someone sleeping on their side or stomach, you will see their buttocks and belly button moving outward on the inhale and relaxing on the exhale.

What can you expect to feel from this breath? Many people feel a warm flush in their face as the breath releases the tension in their bodies. Others report that it feels as though their whole body becomes a sense organ. Still others say it connects their upper and lower chakras. It produces a state of relaxed awareness quite unlike any other breath I have tried.

✳

The Circular Breath

Practice for five to ten minutes.

The essence of the Circular Breath is breathing in a continuous flow, with no break or pause between the inhale and the exhale. The inhale flows effortlessly into the exhale, which flows seamlessly into the next inhale. You can do this breath sitting, standing, or lying down.

1. Breathe gently through your mouth, keeping your jaw relaxed and your lips slightly parted.
2. Feel the back of your throat open and relax. Do not force or push the breath. The inhale will require a bit more effort than the exhale, which should just gently fall out.
3. Imagine your breath making a complete unbroken circle.

This breath is particularly useful for circulating erotic energy around your own body and between yourself and your partner(s). It builds and moves energy, and it intensifies feelings—both emotional and physical.

Some variations on the Circular Breath include breathing in through your nose and out through your mouth, and visualizing an unbroken figure eight instead of a circle.

※
The Breath of Fire

Practice for no longer than one to two minutes.

The Breath of Fire is a Kundalini yoga technique. It is a powerfully energizing breath that gets the little neurons in your brain humming as it clears your lungs and cleanses your blood. The Breath of Fire is aptly named. I usually feel a lot of heat spreading out from the center of my body when I do this breath. This rapid, continuous breath is done entirely through the nose. It can be done in any position, but it's best learned standing or sitting up with a straight spine. The emphasis of this breath is on the exhale.

1. Exhale. As you exhale, push the air out by rapidly pulling your navel to your spine.
2. To inhale, simply release your navel outward. The breath fills your lungs automatically.
3. Put your hand on your diaphragm to focus your attention there and to feel the power of this breath.
4. Begin with one breath every two seconds; work up to one or two breaths per second.

I use the Breath of Fire whenever I want to build energy. This could be at any time before or during sex. It also wakes me up and brings my attention back if I've started to space out. A couple of minutes of this breath is also a great substitute for the caffeine and sugar we start to crave at around 4 p.m. A writer friend of mine uses the Breath of Fire to focus on a particularly difficult passage she might be working on.

※
The Heart Breath

Practice for five to ten minutes.

If you never learn or practice any other kind of breathing (which would be a shame, but I know some people are minimalists), you could have a perfectly lovely time with this one alone. You can speed it up or slow it way down. You can take in a lot of air with a minimum amount of effort and tension. It's a great all-around breath for all erotic purposes. This is the breath we used at the beginning of this chapter, when we first explored how changing our breathing could change our consciousness.

1. Yawn. Feel how the yawn opens the back of your throat and stretches out your whole mouth and face? That's the feeling of openness you want when you do the Heart Breath.
2. Breathe. Let your mouth fall open slightly. Relax your jaw and face, open the back of your throat, and breathe in through your mouth, gently but fully.
3. Exhale. Don't push the breath out; just let it fall out with a gentle little sigh, *ahh*.
4. Take in a much air as you can, as effortlessly as you can, then let it go.
5. Keep breathing.

After you've become familiar with these four conscious breaths and how they make you feel, add sex. Try the breaths while you masturbate. Alternate them. Notice the different effects each one has on the ebb and flow of your erotic energy. You may notice that it will take you longer to reach orgasm while you are doing any or all these conscious breaths. This is good! It means that your breath is moving your sexual energy all over your body. When we masturbate by holding our breath and bearing down (the classic quickie), we limit our sexual energy to the area around our genitals. When we breathe fully and consciously, it's like filling a five-gallon jug instead of a coffee cup. It takes longer, but the payoff is a bigger, deeper, longer orgasm and a more delicious afterglow.

Breathing consciously simply means being mindful, aware, and attentive to your breath. Remember, we can only focus on one thought at a time. If we keep our mind full with our breathing, we don't have the space to think things like "I'll never come," "I wonder if they really love me," or "Did I mail that bill?" Now, I'm not suggesting that you only think about your breath when you have sex. But if you focus on your breath as you might in meditation—that is, using breath as the technique that allows you to actually arrive at the place of meditation—you'll find you're well on your way to conscious sex.

Meditation

When we think of meditation, we usually imagine someone sitting quietly, focusing on their breathing, perhaps chanting *om* or gazing into the flame of a candle. They are blissfully unaware of anything except an exquisite silence punctuated by flashes of inspiring spiritual insight. But, as anyone who has ever meditated knows, the process of meditation is more commonly an exercise in *trying* to meditate. That is, trying to gently pry the mind away from the dozens of thoughts that demand its attention and direct it back to the breath, the chant, or the flame.

The spiritual teacher and modern mystic Osho observed that the Westerners who came to his ashram in India in the 1970s to learn meditation could not begin by just sitting. Their minds were too busy. Trying to sit in meditation made them frustrated, depressed, and kind of crazy. So Osho decided to use that craziness of the mind in preparation for meditation. He created active meditations (although called meditations, they were really *preparations* for meditation) that allowed the natural crazy ego busyness of the mind to speak and scream and worry and natter away, until finally the body and mind could come to a place of relaxation and energized awareness. This relaxed, energized awareness is precisely the state we would like to be in when we want to enjoy conscious sex.

I have created two moving meditations inspired by Osho's meditations—the Exhilaration Meditation and the Cathartic Meditation. Both of these meditations are very active. If a total stranger walked in on you while you were doing them, you would appear, if not crazy, then at least very silly. This is a great gift and a wonderful feeling.

The Power of Silliness

Some of my favorite memories of early childhood are of the spells of uncontrollable, screaming giggles that left me rolling on the ground and gasping for breath. Invariably, these gigglegasms were brought on by silliness—either mine or someone else's. Silliness had power when we were children. Not only could it make us feel terrific, it was often contagious and had the potential to reduce even the most dour of adults to occasional spells of ridiculousness themselves. It was divine. Then came junior high and the "No Silliness" rule. Silliness is cute in little kids, but in hormone-stoked adolescents, it apparently takes on a dangerous edge. Adults who once cooed, "Isn't that cute" were now screaming, "That's enough. Sit down, shut up, and stop behaving like an idiot." Stifling as that was, the adult-generated "No Silliness" rule paled in importance to the peer-generated "No Silliness" rule, which was: "Thou shalt never, ever, under any circumstances, do anything that might possibly make you look like a jerk, *especially* in front of a potential mate."

This rule remains important in junior high school to this day. It has such authority and control that it has transcended junior high and clawed its way to power in our high schools, colleges, and adult lives. We will do almost anything to avoid looking silly or ridiculous. And that's not only tragic, it's well, silly. Silliness still has the same power it did when we were kids. It can free us from our illusions of control and self-importance. It expands our minds, our spirituality, and our sex.

It is time to take back our power. It is time not only to allow ourselves to be silly, but also to embrace our silliness, worship it, and infect as many others with it as we can. The Exhilaration Meditation and Cathartic Meditation (as well as many of the exercises in the rest of this book) have huge silliness potential. They may make you feel silly or look silly. This is not a problem; it is a terrific gift. Feeling shy about trying a silly exercise? Try doing it like this: just close your eyes until the feelings produced by your silliness are more enjoyable than your embarrassment. Then open your eyes and see how delightful silliness looks on your partner. It looks just as good on you.

Witnessing

When you do these extended, active meditations, your mind will often explode with thoughts (not the least of which may be, *When will this damn meditation be over?*). That's okay. You cannot shut off your mind. To notice just how busy and stubborn your mind can be, try practicing the technique of witnessing.

When you witness your thoughts, you notice them, but you do not engage them. It's like lying on your back in a meadow on a breezy day and watching the clouds float by. You just notice that there *are* clouds (your thoughts) and what they look like. You don't jump on them and let them take you away. For example, you might find yourself thinking about work. Instead of allowing your mind to spend twenty minutes worrying about what might happen at the office next week, you simply think, *Oh look, another fearful thought about losing my job.* Or you might notice, *Oops, I almost got swept away with that sexual fantasy about Tom.* When we witness, we do not search for the answer to our relationship with Tom. We do not judge our relationship with Tom. We simply observe that we are having a sexual fantasy about Tom. Witnessing is great practice for training the mind to focus at will.

Witnessing can also be useful for creating distance between yourself and your feelings. When I am extremely sad, angry, or fearful, I try to remember that I am not my emotions. I am me and I am safe in the situation no matter how painful it might be. (I love Louise L. Hay, the metaphysical teacher and author. She once taught me, "Whenever you can say 'I am safe,' you are!") Witnessing helps me remember that my thoughts are fueling my emotions. When I can let my painful thoughts glide by without getting sucked into them, I can calm down and get some clarity on the situation. Then I may still choose to continue to cry or scream or run; but I have made the *conscious choice* to do these things, and that feels altogether lighter, easier, and safer. *I am doing the feeling; the feeling is no longer doing me.*

Conscious choices that produce desirable results—that's Tantra. When we make the conscious choice to focus our attention on our breath, our movement, our speaking, our touch, our feelings, and our lover's eyes, we have engaged our minds to help us connect, relax, and let go.

The Exhilaration and Cathartic Meditations

Both of these meditations can provide a powerful attitude adjustment in as little as twenty minutes, although I think you will find that the longer, fifty- to fifty-five-minute are versions even more effective. I suggest you begin with the twenty-minute versions and work your way up to the longer versions, if you feel so inclined.

The Exhilaration Meditation has three segments. The Cathartic Meditation has five. Doing these meditations to music makes them much more fun and focused; plus you don't have to keep track of the time—the change in music signals the next part. Read over the meditations in advance. Once you know the nature of each part of the mediations, you can make your own soundtrack. I have made several versions of varying lengths. You can also use a timer.

❋
Exhilaration Meditation

Wear comfortable, loose clothing, or no clothes at all. Although you can do the meditation with eyes open or closed, I recommend closing your eyes. If you live in a small space and fear that you'll crash into things, simply plant your feet and shake or dance in place.

Part one (five to fifteen minutes). Shake. Begin by making yourself shake. Shake your arms, hands, belly, thighs, legs, and face. Soon you will find that the shaking happens on its own—the shaking shakes you.

Add gibberish. As you continue shaking, make sounds. Start with one repeated syllable, such as *blah, blah, blah, blah, blah* or *yak, yak, yak, yak, yak*. Let the syllables change and multiply until it seems you are speaking a make-believe language. Let the gibberish be fun. Enjoy the feeling of vibrating on the inside and on the outside at the same time.

Part two (five to fifteen minutes). Dance. Dance any way you feel like. Move from your core. You are not at a club—do not be concerned about the way you look.

Add whirling. After you have been dancing for a while (and only if you have not eaten in the past couple of hours) whirl to your left or your right. Keep your eyes open slightly, but let them be unfocused. Start slowly, then speed up. When you begin to feel dizzy, slow down and whirl in the opposite direction, or close your eyes and return to dancing. A little whirling produces a big effect. Whirl sparingly!

Part three (ten to twenty minutes). Keeping your eyes closed, sit or lie down and be still.

Some people feel nauseous when they whirl. If you know this happens to you, simply dance without whirling. If you become uncomfortably nauseous while whirling, proceed to part three and lie on your stomach. Focus on your heartbeat and breathe. The feeling of nausea while whirling usually dissipates with practice.

※
Cathartic Meditation

The Cathartic Meditation is more energetic and chaotic than the Exhilaration Meditation. It is a great way to begin your day. It is also remarkably effective for throwing off the cumulative physical and psychic effects of a workweek in the big city. Just make sure you have a relatively empty stomach. This meditation is best done with eyes closed or wearing a blindfold.

Part one (four to ten minutes). Breathe forcefully and rapidly through the nose, focusing on the exhalation. The inhalation will happen automatically. This is very similar to the Breath of Fire, but in this case your breath can be more chaotic. Allow your body to move with your breath and use those natural body movements to help you build up your energy. The purpose of this part is to build energy that you will release in the next part.

Part two (four to ten minutes). Release your inner two-year-old! Clench your fists and jump up and down while yelling "NO!" with each jump. After several minutes of "NO!" unclench your fists and raise your open hands to shoulder height. Keep jumping, but this time yell "YES!" on each jump. Yell "YES!" with the same force and intensity that you have been yelling "NO!"

Part three (four to ten minutes). Release your inner kung fu fighter. Stand in a power stance with knees bent and feet a bit more than shoulder distance apart. Tilt your pelvis back and tighten your abdominal muscles and your buttocks until you feel strong and invincible. Now throw karate chops in front of you, releasing a powerful karate yell with each karate chop.

Part four (four to fifteen minutes). Stop! Immediately place your body in a manageable sitting or standing pose and then do not move. Do not rearrange your body, just let it be. Focus on your breath or on your heartbeat. Simply witness whatever happens.

Part five (four to ten minutes). Laugh. Begin with a smile. Let the smile grow wider until it becomes a giggle. Let the giggle grow until it becomes laughter. Then let the laughing laugh you. Become laughter.

You can do the Cathartic Meditation without risking eviction for noise violations with these modifications: in part two, yell "NO!" and then "YES" silently inside yourself; and in part three, you can throw karate chops with a sharp exhale instead of a yell.

There are other simple and very effective cathartic meditations. One is pillow beating. If you are feeling angry at someone or something, beat a pillow. If you let your pillow thrashing be a meditation, the anger will turn into a kind of energy phenomenon. You may feel silly, you may feel sad, you may feel elated. You may even have an angergasm. Whatever happens, the anger will be transformed and you will feel calmer and more centered.

> ## The Silent Scream
>
> If you just need to scream and you live in a building where that will produce a call to 911, try screaming underwater. Fill your bathtub with nice warm water, get in, put your face in the water, and scream away. Even someone in the next room probably won't hear you. And you'll feel so much better. (Just remember not to inhale while your head is underwater.)

These active mediations will not eliminate *all* of your negative feelings. That's fine. You don't *need* to eliminate all negative feelings in order to make love consciously. Heck, if we all waited to have sex until we felt perfectly blissful, we'd never fuck at all! What active meditations will do for you is open you up and relax you so that your feelings are not so stuck and binding. When your energy is flowing and your mind is quiet, it doesn't matter so much *what* you are feeling; it only matters that you *are* feeling. And remember: feeling *silly* is a perfectly lovely doorway to feeling *sexy*.

Even a short active meditation will sensitize not only your emotional body but also your physical body. You may notice that you have more feeling in your hands or in parts of your body that seemed numb before you did the meditation. This alive, awake, sensitive state is ideal for learning and practicing a kind of touching that can make your insides melt. Let's explore the deep deliciousness of conscious touch.

CHAPTER 5

How to Touch

Sex, whether Tantric or not, involves touch. Lots of touch. Traditional sex guides usually discuss which body part to touch, when to touch it, and how fast to touch it. This is great, as far as it goes. But in Tantra, we want to go a step further. We want to *become* the touch. In order to do that, we need to find the narrow realm of touch that lies between too much pressure and too little. When you touch the body, you want to touch deeply enough that the body pushes back just a little. If a muscle becomes rigid under your touch, you've gone too far. If the muscle feels flaccid, you haven't gone far enough.

The Resilient Edge of Resistance

This is the essence of conscious touch. It was named the Resilient Edge of Resistance by my endlessly inventive teaching partner, Chester Mainard. If the concept of the Resilient Edge of Resistance sounds complicated or vague, think about all the times you've been touched. What does it feel like when someone's touch is too tentative? It may feel like an annoying tickle, or—if they are using the tips of their fingers—it may feel like poking. Either way, it feels just plain icky. At the other end of the spectrum, some people's touch is way too intense. Have you ever received a massage by someone with a really heavy touch? Your muscles tense and contract as if trying to push their hands away. You get more and more tense as they try to force your muscles to relax. It is painful and not at all relaxing. Then there's the touch that is just right. It feels safe and supportive and present. It's neither too hard nor too soft. It lulls you into a place of deep comfort and surrender. You're awake and aware, but completely peaceful and relaxed at the same time. You want it to go on forever. The person touching you has found your Resilient Edge of Resistance.

Place your hand on your lower arm very lightly. Don't apply any pressure. Notice what this feels like. Now massage your arm, applying increasingly more pressure. Stop at the point where the massage becomes painful. Notice what this feels like. Now lighten your touch until you find the point at which your arm yields to your touch but does not shrink away from it. You might find it with a massage stroke using your fingers, or just by holding your arm.

I've always thought a good illustration of the edge of resistance is the tummy touch on the Pillsbury doughboy in those television commercials. When the doughboy is touched on his tummy, he absorbs the touch (the finger makes a little dimple on his tummy); then his doughy tummy springs right back, and the doughboy giggles. That's the Resilient Edge of Resistance.

This same dynamic applies to all parts of our being: physical, emotional, and psychic. When we have too much mental stress in our lives, we shut down, overwhelmed; yet when there is too little stress, we have no energy, no motivation. On the psychic level, the Resilient Edge of Resistance translates into "sufficiently supported to take a risk." Without risk, there is no growth or energy; however, without support, risk becomes recklessness. In the territory between, we can grow, thrive, and find pleasure. We function optimally at the Resilient Edge of Resistance.

The Resilient Edge of Resistance shifts constantly. When pressure is applied to the edge of resistance—whether that pressure is breath, touch, or tension—you expand a bit. This creates a new edge of resistance. Yoga postures are a good example of this. If you are seated on the floor and bend over to try to touch your forehead to your legs, it may at first seem impossible. Then, with each breath, you relax into the stretch a little bit more. You don't force it, you just open up a bit more with each breath. Before you know it, your nose is a lot closer to your legs than you ever thought possible. By staying at the Resilient Edge of Resistance, you are able to go much deeper into the pose than if you had not gone to the edge, or if you had pushed past the edge into pain. The Resilient Edge of Resistance is the place where you feel safe enough to surrender and go deeper.

Sex that is too soft is vapid; sex that is too hard is assaulting. We want to learn to dance on the Resilient Edge of Resistance because that's where the real pleasure is. When we reach that level of pleasure, gateways open to even more profound discoveries and connections.

Most people touch the way they like to be touched, which may not be how someone else likes to be touched at all. For example, you may go all melty and shivery when someone lightly runs their fingernails along the inside of your thighs. Quite naturally, you'll want your partner to feel as yummy as you do, so you'll touch him the same way. However, he may find that light, feathery touch ticklish and annoying. So how do you learn to recognize the Resilient Edge of Resistance? Your hands and your intuition will guide you, but your best guide is the person you are touching. Ask your partner to tell you when a touch is too hard or too light. When you get feedback, you can easily make an adjustment, and your hands will memorize it. With practice, your hands will know what the Resilient Edge of Resistance feels like on more and more places on the body, and your touch will become as perfect as that of the lady whose fingertip poked the tummy of the Pillsbury doughboy.

Here are a few exercises to help you write the Resilient Edge of Resistance into your muscle memory:

* Hug someone. Find a connection that is neither too smothering nor too wimpy.
* Set the temperature of your bath or shower water to the point where any hotter would be too hot and any colder would be too cold.
* Give yourself a massage with body cream. Go slowly and find the Resilient Edge of Resistance on your legs, your arms, your belly, and your breasts.
* Give and receive a hand massage.
* Get a massage. Explain the concept of the Resilient Edge of Resistance to your masseuse. With her agreement, give feedback to keep the masseuse's touch at your edge.
* Give a massage. Ask the receiver to give you feedback to keep your touch at their Resilient Edge of Resistance.
* Practice by petting a cat or a dog. Pets give great feedback. If they stick around and beg for more, you've found their Resilient Edge of Resistance.
* Find the Resilient Edge of Resistance in stillness. Stillness is extremely powerful. Put your hands on someone so that you can feel both resilience and resistance. Embrace them with your hands.

The Resilient Edge of Resistance Applies to More Than Touch

Although the Resilient Edge of Resistance is a concept most easily applied to touch, all of your relating with a lover (including yourself) can take place in the lovely realm between too much pressure and too little. Let me give you an example. Several years ago, I met my adorable and adoring partner, Kate, at a most intense time in my life. I was breaking up with one lover, involved with two others in a three-way, long-distance relationship, and packing up my New York City home to move to Australia. Not a day went by that I wasn't saying goodbye to someone or something that had been a hugely important part of my life. The stress was high as an elephant's eye, and I was starting to crack under the pressure and grief and drama of it all.

One afternoon, Kate and I started to make love. She was touching me lightly and lovingly, and it should have been wonderful, but it wasn't. I couldn't stand it—I wanted to punch her. Of course, it wasn't her fault. I usually loved a light, elegant touch. After all, I was the queen of ostrich feather caresses and silky, sensuous massages. But today it just wasn't working for me at all. Kate, both a very experienced S/M player and a very intuitive lover, said, "Do you think you might like something a little harder?"

"Definitely."

She began by thudding my back with a padded nightstick. It felt so good. I breathed and groaned and yelled out weeks of built-up pain and frustration. When I turned over, I felt a tight pain in my solar plexus as though some malevolent force had grabbed hold of all my power and was holding it hostage. Kate took a sharp, pointed talon (a long steel claw that extends from a ring worn on the finger to an inch beyond the fingertip) and started running it down my stomach. She started relatively lightly, as the talon was quite sharp. I kept asking her to press harder and harder. With each stroke I was opening up a bit more. Kate stayed right with me. She listened to me, gave me what I asked for, and, most important, made me feel safe. I knew she was focused only on me and that she had the technique to use the talon safely. I knew she would not do anything that would actually injure me, no matter how much I asked. I breathed and yelled and cried, and finally, as the talon nearly sliced me open, I felt my solar plexus burst open, releasing all the evil, black, psychic gunk I had been holding there. I cried and cried and then I laughed and laughed. I felt so high, so light, and so me again.

That was meeting the Resilient Edge of Resistance—psychically, emotionally, and physically. So, think about your own life: where you live, what you do for work, what your home life is like, and so forth. If you live in a sweet little cottage beside a lake in the woods, work at a fulfilling but low-pressure job, and have lots of time for family and friends and nature, your Resilient Edge of Resistance will be at a very different place at the end of a day than that of a person who works in a cubicle in a corporate office tower in midtown New York at a high-pressure job that frequently keeps them at their desk till 9 p.m. The person in New York is more likely to want and need a harder touch in order to crack through the armor they have built up to protect their hearts and other soft tender parts. Whether you generally like a hard touch or a soft touch, whether you like black leather or floaty sarongs, even if you change your sexual style on a daily basis, you can't go wrong if you simply find your Resilient Edge of Resistance.

CHAPTER 6

Twenty-Minute Tantra

Perhaps you're beginning to think, *Good grief, if I have to meditate and then practice new ways to breathe and touch, when will I ever have time for sex? There's just not enough time!* I understand completely. I often fall into the there's-never-enough-time trap, especially when I've got twice as many things to do as I have hours in which to do them. Time itself feels like a rare and precious resource that's always just about to run dry. I also feel guilty about the time I "waste" when I sleep an extra hour. And I also fantasize about all the things I could accomplish if only there were a couple more hours in the day. It seems we're all either falling behind or racing to catch up.

However, this does not have to be just one more self-help book you skim through and then leave on the shelf because you never had enough time to try any of the things you read. Tantra can be learned and practiced in the time you actually have.

But first, you need to understand that you do have *some* time. Time is not a fixed, inflexible commodity. If it were, each day would seem exactly the same length as the one before. We know that isn't the case—some days feel endless while others zip by in an instant. Time is malleable. Time is part of us; it belongs to us; it's something we have power to control. There is a good reason why we *feel* so powerless over time: we give so much of it away to everything and everyone else that there simply isn't much left for ourselves. Consistently putting the things we "should" do and "must" do ahead of the things we "could" do and "want to" do is exhausting, depleting, depressing, and completely libido-dampening.

The media is full of reports of people in committed relationships who aren't having sex. This is not the same old story of men who want more sex than their wives. Now, more and more wives are complaining that their husbands are the ones who don't want sex. People often say their dearth of sexual activity is because they just don't have time. But is that the truth? Is it really *time* that we are lacking?

The statement "I don't have the time for sex" usually has little to do with time *or* sex. More often, it means "I'm tired," or "I really need to work," or "I'd really *rather* work." It can mean "I want to spend more time with the children" or "I have spent way, way too much time with the children." It often means "I need some time completely to myself—away from everything and everyone. I have nothing left to give." Our desire for sex (especially for partner sex) can be depleted by, among other things, anxiety, depression, antidepressants, lack of work, overwork, or even an obsession with our children. It's not that we don't have the time for sex, it's just that other things seem more important, necessary, or enjoyable than sex. Ironically, sex is probably just the thing to alleviate the depression, exhaustion, anxiety, and obsession.

Instead of saying that we want more time for sex, I think we'd be more truthful saying that we want *better* time—time with no looming concerns or commitments. Many of us neither need nor want vast expanses of free time. Vast, empty periods of time can be daunting, especially when filled with long silences as we try to express our craving for sex or the kind of intimacy we experience through sex. One of the most effective tricks we use to avoid sex or intimacy is the excuse "I just don't have time right now. Let's talk about it later."

How do we solve this time/sex/intimacy conundrum? We start small. We select small amounts of time and the kinds of sexual activities that can be exciting and satisfying in a short period of time. Please, don't wait until there's time for a five-hour Tantric ritual. You may never find those five hours. Don't even wait until you are "in the mood." There are sexy things you can do that will increase your desire. You can start practicing Tantra in whatever mood you are in. You only need twenty minutes.

Conscious Quickies

Twenty minutes? What can you do with twenty minutes? Plenty.

* It was a twenty-minute lap dancing session with that cowboy that resulted in my mind-blowing flight through the cosmos.
* Even if you're feeling too tired for sex, twenty minutes of selfloving can put you into a lovely, deep, peaceful sleep.
* In twenty minutes, you can easily give yourself an energy orgasm that will leave you emotionally and physically refreshed.
* Both the Exhilaration Meditation and Cathartic Meditation can be accomplished in twenty minutes.

Stop thinking in hours, days, and weekends, and start thinking twenty minutes. A week of juicy, twenty-minute conscious quickies once a day will add up to two and one-half hours of sex per week. By the way, if your partner does not want to participate in your conscious quickies, that's okay. There are plenty of techniques that you can practice alone. Remember, you are doing conscious quickies for *you*. You're not trying to trick or trap your partner(s) into doing anything they really don't want to do. However, you may find that your partner(s) are increasingly likely to join you if you are consistent and dedicated to your daily twenty minutes.

Think of sex as an art, like music or painting. Becoming accomplished in any art takes regular practice. Any music teacher will tell you that twenty minutes of practice every day is more effective than two and a half hours once a week. Why? Because the body is an instrument that responds well to steady, consistent repetition. Whether you want your body to dance a solo, play a sonata, or be capable of multiple full-body orgasms, you need the kind of practice that's going to get you results. Unconsciously jerking off to a porn magazine certainly will not hurt you, but it won't improve your technique or increase your capacity for more pleasure, either. The kind of practice I'm talking about is *conscious* practice. No matter how scattered your thoughts or how busy your life, you certainly can keep your attention focused on an erotic exercise for twenty minutes.

Your conscious quickies will open up all the pathways through which sexual energy flows in your body so you will become more aroused and erotically charged in less and less time. When you develop a steady sexual practice, you'll look forward to the practice more and more. You may find yourself happily doing more than twenty minutes per day.

And when you are looking forward to sex and erotic pleasure, please remember that sex does not always have to be mind-blowing. It can be quiet and soft and comforting. It can be sad or angry or scary. Let go of any expectations or goals you may have regarding what you will "achieve" in your conscious quickies. Release your performance anxiety, don't try to be perfect, learn to improvise, and experiment a little, even when you are not in the mood. Use your conscious quickies to tune your erotic instrument.

The exercises in this book are designed to help you increase your awareness, your energy, and your capacity for pleasure. They will help you to return to your natural state as a human *being*—as opposed to the human *doing* you may have become. Many, if not most, of the exercises can be done as conscious quickies: twenty-minute erotic adventures that you can have alone or with others. When you have more time, you'll be able to weave your favorite exercises together into your own yummy ritual.

A word of caution: we've all been told a thousand times that to achieve a happier, more pleasure-filled life, we must begin by putting ourselves first. Well, that may be true, but with the pressures of work, family, school, children, parents, and partners, it can be difficult to find ourselves on our own priority list. Just think of your conscious quickies as twenty magical minutes that nourish you and still leave you with twenty-three hours and forty minutes to handle everything else. After you've spent twenty deeply conscious minutes pleasing yourself, the rest *will* be easier to handle.

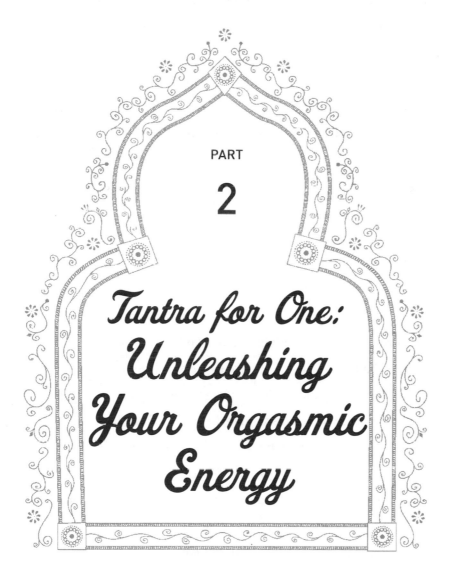

PART

2

Tantra for One: Unleashing Your Orgasmic Energy

Jwala, my first Tantra teacher, is fond of asking her workshop participants to list ten qualities they would want in their ideal lover. She doesn't mean physical qualities like big breasts or sculpted abs. The qualities she wants you to list are things like enthusiasm, kindness, or having a twisted sense of humor.

Try it if you like. Stop reading after the end of the next sentence, and make your own list. When you've finished, continue on to the next paragraph.

Read over your list. Does this person remind you of anyone you already know?

Chances are, you have done a pretty good job of describing yourself. Most people do. And that's perfect. After all, you are the one love who will never leave you. You'll always want sex when you do. You'll always know exactly how to please you. And your parents would probably even approve of your choice.

So now that we know who your ideal lover is, let the romance begin! This chapter will show you how to activate and channel your sexual energy into all sorts of delightful orgasmic adventures. You'll even enter the amazing world of breath and chakra orgasms—full-body orgasms you can achieve simply by breathing. You'll get to try all sorts of new sensations as you discover what truly turns you on. Finally, you'll take yourself out on a Tantric date.

Tantra for one is not simply what you do when you can't get a date with someone else. Solo Tantra is the lifelong process of falling in love and staying in love with yourself—not just sexually, but also in respect, devotion, and compassion. Along the path, you may just discover that you've attracted one or more other delightful beings who love you just as much as you love yourself.

CHAPTER 7

Sexual Energy: What It Is and What to Do with It

In Tantra, sex is not an action. It is not one more thing humans *do*. Sex is an energy that exists on its own. All you have to do is notice it and it will start to move. But what exactly is sexual energy? Is it the feeling you get in your genitals when you're aroused? Is it the sexual desire you feel for someone? Is it the warm, loving feeling you have for your beloved?

The first step toward getting in touch with your sexual energy is to actually feel that energy. Sexual energy is an actual physical energy, not just a desire, a thought, or an emotion. Let me show you what I mean. Try this: rub your hands together vigorously for about ten seconds. Stop and hold your hands together so that the palms are not quite touching. Feel that hot little force field running between your two hands? You've just created energy in your hands using movement—in this case, you used friction.

Now rub your hands together again. Feel the energy between your hands. Put your hands on your heart and send the energy into your heart. Breathe. Does your heart feel warmer? Are you more aware of it?

You have just used intention and movement to create energy in one part of your body and send it to another. This is the first step to making your whole body a sex organ.

But was the energy you just created *sexual* energy? Sure. There isn't any difference between sexual energy and creative energy, or between sexual energy and going-to-work energy, or between sexual energy and taking-out-the-trash energy. It's all life-force energy.

There is nothing mysterious about moving sexual energy around the body—yours or someone else's. Anybody can do it. You don't have to be psychic; you don't need to attend any channeling workshops. You did it just now with movement, touch, and thought. Tantra is filled with numerous ingenious ways to build, circulate, and use sexual energy. Let's explore some of them now.

Kundalini, Chi, and the Inner Flute

In yogic—including Tantric—tradition, our sexual energy is called Kundalini. It is depicted as a coiled snake resting at the base of our spine. With conscious practice, we awaken this snake of energy sleeping at the first chakra, and it spirals up along the spine, flowing through two channels (called the Ida and Pingala), passing through each chakra, and finally activating the pineal gland at the seventh chakra. When the pineal gland is activated, a major change in consciousness is experienced. Yogis see Kundalini as the energy of human evolution and enlightenment and warn that if Kundalini is awakened too soon or too abruptly, it can cause serious difficulties. That's how powerful a force it is.

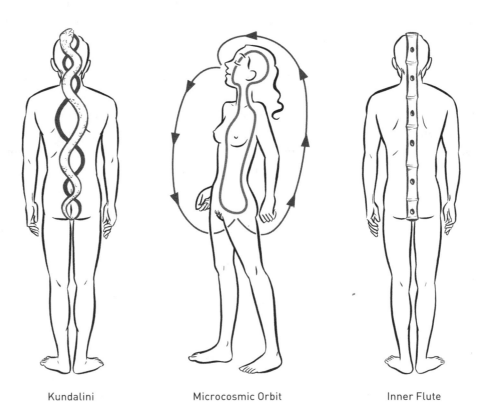

Kundalini   Microcosmic Orbit   Inner Flute

In the Chinese Taoist tradition, life-force energy is called *chi*. Sexual energy is called *ching-chi*. Chi travels in a big electrical circuit called the Microcosmic Orbit. The Microcosmic Orbit is made up of two channels: the back (Governor Channel) and the front (Functional Channel). The back channel begins at the perineum and runs up the back of the body. It follows the spine and neck up over the top of the head and down the forehead, ending at the indentation between the bottom of your nose and your upper lip. The front channel runs from the tip of your tongue, down your throat, and along the midline of the front of your body to your perineum. In this tradition, letting energy flow down the front channel is equally important as raising it up the spine. This flow of energy acknowledges the peculiar nature of being human: we are both bodies rising toward spirit and spirits dropping into bodies.

Yet another Taoist-based tradition speaks of the Inner Flute, an energetic (nonphysical) tube that runs up through the core of the body connecting the major endocrine glands and the seven chakras. I like to picture the body as a bamboo flute—all the flesh, bones, and blood are part of the bamboo. The bamboo is hollow—inside is just empty space. Sexual energy runs up and down the body through this bamboo flute, as you'll see for yourself when you use the Taoist-based breath and energy orgasm technique called the Clench and Hold (see chapter 9).

There are many other names for this energy of sex and life force. Each tradition has its own name and its own way of working with it. Many practices, across many cultures, are virtually indistinguishable. Differences in details make for subtle and fascinating variations on the themes. Here, we will work primarily with the terminology and traditions of Tantra and Tao. However, I encourage you to go beyond the exercises and suggestions in this book. Follow the lead of the energy you raise in your sexual explorations and create your own practices, traditions, and rituals.

"Seeing" Sexual Energy

Sexual energy is extraordinarily visible on the body. With a little practice, you'll be able to read and interpret the signs and observe how it moves. For instance, earlier we were talking about moving energy up the chakras. Is there any way to see that energy move? Let's say you are eagerly sucking and licking your partner's clit. At the same time, you are using your hands to spread all that yummy sexual energy up to her breasts and down her arms. You're curious about how and where that sexual energy is moving. Unless your partner is someone like me, who is fascinated by the physical technology of sacred sex, it's probably not appropriate to ask, "Honey, what chakra are we up to?" So how can you tell?

One way is to listen to the sounds she is making. Is the sound low pitched and sort of grunty/groany? If it is, the energy is concentrated in the lower chakras. If the sound is breathy, mid-pitched, and sounds like *ahh*, the sexual energy has moved up to the heart and throat chakras. If it is high pitched and sounds like *eee*, then the sexual energy is dancing around the third eye or crown chakra.

But sound isn't the only way to tell where sexual energy is concentrated. As energy moves up the body, the body moves with it. When you first start to suck your lover's clit, she may begin by bumping and grinding her hips. Then she may do little back bend–like motions, raising her solar plexus, or heart chakra, into the air. She may end up shaking her head or throwing it backward as the energy reaches her upper chakras. As you shift your intention and attention away from "doing" sex and more toward dancing to the energy of sex, you'll become more and more aware of how sexual energy moves and travels throughout the body.

Dropping into the Body

This is a probably a good time to dispel a common misconception. It often sounds as if the goal in "higher" sex practices is to raise the energy out of the genitals upward into the higher chakras until we shoot our consciousness out the tops of our heads—which somehow sounds like a "higher" kind of sexual experience than one that happens in the genitals. This is exactly the kind of body-negative thinking that we would like to change.

We *do* want to bring sexual energy up and out into the entire body. But we do *not* bring sexual energy up into the higher chakras in order to take it away from the lower chakras. There is nothing "better" about the higher chakras. Nor are the chakras a stepladder leading sexual energy out of the body into some special, more spiritual realm. We do not want to shoot ourselves out of our bodies; rather, we want to drop into our bodies more deeply and completely.

For hundreds of years, organized religions have regarded the body as something we must overcome with strict spiritual practices. Even today, some New Age spiritual practices use meditation as an attempt to leave the body for a "higher state" of consciousness.

The intention is not to leave the body,

but to drop into the body more deeply and completely.

We are at our healthiest when we are circulating energy both within ourselves and within our relationships. Energy is the basic building block of all human creativity and connection. Sexual energy flows through all our creative and social endeavors: work, sports, money, birth, death, friendships, and all family relationships, including parent/child. The connection we have to all other living beings through the erotic energy field is natural and healthy. When your sexual energy is flowing freely, you feel alive and connected. When it's blocked, you feel dead and lifeless. Every movement is an effort. You may actually feel as though parts of yourself are missing. Connecting with someone else, perhaps even a simple phone conversation, is just too hard. Of course, that kind of lifelessness may be caused by a *lack* of energy, but it can just as likely be a product of some dense, tightly bound-up energy stuck somewhere in your body between your genitals and the top of your head.

Try this: Close your eyes (*after* you've finished reading this paragraph, naturally). Turn your attention inward. Notice which parts of your physical body you can feel. Can you feel your feet, legs, genitals, belly, spine, arms, hands, throat, head, eyes, and mouth? What parts aren't there at all? Which are shadowy and vague?

This exercise may help you get some idea of where your energy might be stuck. Breath is a great tool to use to begin to get energy moving again. Breath is the source of the body's oxygen. Oxygen helps each cell burn fuel at maximum efficiency, thereby producing more energy. The simple act of using your mind to direct your breath into the sleeping parts of your body will begin to wake them up.

But sometimes, breath alone just isn't enough to shake loose a week's worth of tension and bring you back to your cheerful, yummy self. I put together the following series of exercises to help me clear out old, stuck energy blocks and get my energy flowing again. Sometimes I do one or two of the exercises, sometimes the whole series. Sometimes I do each exercise only once, or maybe twice. Sometimes I'll repeat an exercise over and over. Sometimes when I do these exercises I come to realize what in my body had become stuck, and why; most times I don't need to know.

Doing these exercises will break up your energy blocks and improve your mood considerably.

❊
Eye Circles

When your field of vision is wider and more relaxed, you can see more possibilities and opportunities for pleasure and growth. Eye circles help to relax your upper facial muscles and literally open up your eyes. (However, be careful not to force any of the following eye movements.)

1. Lie on your back with your eyes open, looking at the ceiling or sky. Breathe.
2. Moving only your eyes, not your head:
   a) Look to the right as far as you can.
   b) Look down toward your feet.
   c) Look to the left as far as you can.
   d) Look up and behind you as far as you can.
3. Notice how much you can see at each point.
4. Repeat, connecting the four points into a slow circle.
5. Repeat the circle.
6. Circle three times in the opposite direction.

Did your field of vision increase? Were you able to see more and further than when you started?

❊
Jaw Massage

We all carry tension in our jaws. Many of us carry so much tension that we talk through clenched teeth or even grind our teeth. When our jaws are relaxed, all our creative expression flows more easily. Not only do we speak decisively and lovingly, we are also more able to express ourselves sexually.

1. Breathe.
2. Massage your jaw.
3. While massaging, make sounds. Any sounds. Be silly.
4. Massage the joint where your jaw joins your head.
5. Holding your jaw in your hands, wiggle it from side to side.
6. Place your fingers on your lips and cheeks, and massage your teeth and gums.

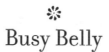

Head Rolls

Our necks are like huge railroad switching stations. All the messages traveling from our brains to our bodies (and vice versa) pass through this narrow, busy station on their way to their destination. When our neck muscles tense up like steel bands, the energy passes through the neck slowly. It's painful and difficult. When our neck muscles are relaxed, the energy flows smoothly and regularly. You feel better and you feel more.

1. Breathe.
2. Allow your head to fall to the right only as far as it wants to go. Do not force it. Let your breath and gravity guide you.
3. Roll your head around in a circle from the right, down to your chest and around to your left shoulder.
4. Let your head fall backward (gently), and then roll it back to the right.
5. Repeat.
6. Circle in the opposite direction.
7. Repeat until your neck feels longer and softer.

Busy Belly

The prevailing cultural preference for flat-as-a-board abdomens encourages people to walk around with tightly sucked-in bellies. Sucking in your belly cuts off sexual feelings in the pelvis and prevents sexual energy from rising up through your body. This exercise will help you free up your belly and allow your natural juiciness to flow.

1. Begin on your hands and knees.
2. As you inhale, fill your belly with your breath. Make your belly as big as you can. Your spine will arch slightly, but don't force it. (If it hurts or you feel a lot of tension, you're forcing it.) Keep your focus on making your belly big, not on arching your spine.
3. As you exhale, draw your belly up into your ribs and spine as far as you can. Your spine will bow slightly. Again, keep your focus on sucking in your belly—not on curving your spine.
4. Repeat as many times as feels good.

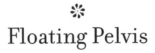

Bouncing Pelvis

Our tendency to suck in our bellies also creates a strain on our lower backs. The lower back is also the repository for the tension we create when we worry about money and security. This exercise loosens up the lower back and wakes up that powerful, sexy Kundalini snake at the base of your spine.

This exercise should be done on a well-carpeted floor or on an exercise mat.

1.   Lie on your back, with your arms by your sides and your palms facing downward.
2.   Bend your knees and bring your feet comfortably close to your buttocks.
3.   Lift your hips off the ground and bounce your buttocks on the floor. Begin gently and intensify the bouncing as your buttocks, lower spine, and genitals relax. Take care not to hurt your lower spine!

Floating Pelvis

Alternate the Bouncing Pelvis with the Floating Pelvis.

1.   After some bouncing, lift your hips off the ground and "float" them in a figure eight.
2.   Alternate bouncing and floating as long as it feels good.

As you work with these exercises, you'll probably find a favorite, which will likely be focused on the chakra or body part where you hold most of your tension. My favorite is the bouncing/floating combination, as I tend to store all my tension in my lower back. That pelvic combination really loosens me up. When time is tight (and when isn't it?), a couple of minutes of bouncing and floating, and I'm good to go again. So, find the one or two of these exercises you can rely on, and use them whenever you want to feel more alive and connected.

As you begin to notice which exercise appeals to you most, also notice the corresponding chakra. Then find out more about that chakra. Start by taking another look at the discussion of that chakra in chapter 3. Research that chakra in other books or on the Internet (see the resources section at the end of the book for suggestions). See if you can find other ways to nourish that chakra. As we go along, you'll find specific ways you can use sex and sexual energy to stimulate and nurture any of the chakras and their corresponding body parts that need special healing.

Let's Dance

Now that you've loosened up the places in your body most likely to accumulate tension, let's start running some sexual energy. Everyone has a personal metaphor for sex. Some think of it as a sport, others as play, and others as a meditation. I think of sex as a dance. Sometimes it's a solo piece, sometimes it's a pas de deux, and sometimes it's a whole ballet. Bodies are meant to be in motion. In fact, bodies are always in motion, if only on the inside. Your beating heart, your breathing lungs, and your digestion all happen to an internal beat.

I learned an especially valuable lesson on this rhythm of life when I studied with jazz dancer and dance teacher Luigi (his only name, like Cher). At the height of his career as a dancer in 1940s Hollywood, Luigi was paralyzed in a near-fatal car crash. He described looking out from inside his silent, frozen body and knowing with complete certainty that if he didn't keep moving, he would die. So, deep inside his body, he found something he could move, and he kept it moving. He moved more and more parts of his body like this until eventually he could move enough to begin doing dance exercises. These movement exercises not only brought him back to health, but to dance as well. Three years later, he was dancing in films with Gene Kelly and Donald O'Connor.

Every move Luigi taught his students came from what he had learned in his rehabilitation. During these jazz dance classes, I could feel each move I'd make start deep within my abdomen and extend out infinitely. It was a feeling of extraordinary and ecstatic power. Ever since then, I have tried to move using that model. Paradoxically, I also learned from Luigi how to practice total stillness. The secret? Keep moving in place. Try it. You cannot stand perfectly still if you tense up and try not to move. After a few brief moments you'll start to sway. But if you relax, breathe, and keep moving inside, you'll be perfectly still on the outside. Bodies need to be in motion—to stand perfectly still involves countless little movements to keep the balance that is stillness.

So what does all this have to do with sex? Simple: you need to move in order to circulate erotic energy throughout your body. Movement in any part of your body focuses and releases energy from that part. Then the energy can be spread to any other part. Which movements work best? Just as in jazz dance, it's those that come from the hips and pelvis. Let's start with simple hip circles.

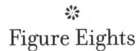

Hip Circles

1. Stand with your feet hip-distance apart.
2. Swing your hips to the right as far as you can without putting strain on your lower back.
3. Now push your pelvis forward.
4. Swing your hips to the left.
5. Now push your buttocks as far back as you can. Remember, be kind to your back.
6. Connect those four points in a smooth circle.
7. Repeat a few times, and then circle in the opposite direction.

Figure Eights

Now let's try some figure eights. Close your eyes, imagine yourself a belly dancer in some exotic temple, and let go.

1. Move your hips in a figure-eight motion. (Swing your hips back-right-front on the right side, then back-left-front on the left side.)
2. Remember that this isn't an aerobics class—this is sex. Let it be sexy. This is a perfect time to add some Kegels.

Kegels

Kegels are your own personal erotic energy pumps. A Kegel is a little squeeze of the pubococcygeus (or PC) muscle. To find that muscle, imagine that you are in the bathroom peeing and someone unexpectedly opens the bathroom door. What do you do? You stop peeing. Feel that? That little muscle that stopped the flow of urine? Squeezing that muscle constitutes a Kegel—named for Dr. Arnold Kegel (pronounced *kay*-gull), a gynecologist who developed a program for women who were experiencing incontinence after giving birth. But in reality, these little squeezes have been known by many names as integral parts of sexual fitness and pleasure for centuries. And they are just as important for men as they are for women. But let's stop talking and let's start Kegeling.

1. Gently squeeze the PC muscle for a couple of seconds. Release.
2. Again, squeeze, and release.
3. Repeat for a total of eight Kegels.
4. Do eight Kegels as fast as you can.

Remember to be gentle. If you're doubling over with each squeeze, you're working too hard!

Don't worry if it feels as if you are also tightening your anus when you Kegel. This isn't a problem. But as you strengthen your PC muscle, you'll probably notice that you can isolate it more and more from the surrounding muscles of the pelvic floor.

The PC muscle is a critically important sexual muscle. For men, the squeezing and tightening in Kegels will help achieve stronger erections. For women, toning your sexual muscle will enhance your vagina's sensitivity and responsiveness, as well as your ability to shoot your sexual energy out all over your body. If you enjoy vaginal penetration with a penis, you will eventually be able to keep a penis erect inside you just by squeezing your PC muscle.

Try to do one hundred to two hundred Kegels per day. You can do Kegels anywhere: standing in line at the bank, waiting for the traffic light to change, walking down the street, or working out at the gym. And they will certainly keep you from nodding off in those boring business meetings. No one but you will know you are doing your erotic exercises.

❀

The Wave

You can add Kegels to the next exercise, called the Wave. I learned the Wave from my friend Kutira. Kutira is a Tantra teacher who lives in Hawaii and swims with dolphins. This exercise is an easy, erotic, and effective way to move sexual energy around. Try it.

1. Stand with your feet hip-distance apart.
2. Bend your knees slightly.
3. Imagine you are an ocean wave, or a dolphin.
4. Swing your pelvis forward and let the rest of your torso follow. As your breastbone moves forward and up, your back arches. This is the top of the wave.
5. Round your shoulders and your back; your pelvis swings back.
6. Swing your pelvis forward and let the rest of your torso follow.
7. Repeat.

Erotically urgent:

Did you remember to breathe during these sexercises?

❋
Put It All Together

Over and over again in Tantra, we will be using a combination of breath, Kegels, movement, awareness, and imagination to build and circulate sexual energy. Let's use the Wave to practice combining these elements. It's easier than you might think.

1. Put on some music you'd like to move to. Make sure it's something that makes you want to move your hips.
2. Stand with your feet hip-distance apart. Bend your knees slightly.
3. Breathe. Let your mouth fall open slightly. Relax your jaw and face, open the back of your throat. Inhale through your mouth, gently but fully. Exhale with a gentle little sigh . . . ahh.
4. Begin the Wave. Start gently, and let it build.
5. Add a Kegel to each wave. You decide where it goes in your wave. There is no right or wrong place to add it.
6. Put your awareness in your genitals. Each time you Kegel, imagine sexual energy being released from your genitals and carried up the front of your body by your breath. At the top of your wave, your sexual energy moves over the top of your head and down your back to your genitals again. Keep yourself wrapped in a cocoon of sexual energy. (Some people feel the wave of energy move up their back and down their front. That's perfectly fine.)
7. Keep breathing, keep the Wave going, and keep the Kegels going. Let it be sexy.
8. Now, instead of "doing" the breath, the Wave, and the Kegels, let them all "do" you. Let the energy you've built move you in any way it wants to. Just go with it and have fun!

Now that you know the basic ways in which sexual energy moves in the body, let's put this knowledge to good use. Let's have some orgasms.

CHAPTER 8

Orgasm: The Totality of Possibilities

I was listening to my local National Public Radio station; an interview was in progress with a sociologist who had written a new book. The big problem in society today, she claimed, was that we had gotten sex all wrong. Sex was not about pleasure, it was about reproduction and producing children. What was the biggest single mistake we had all made? We were all putting too much emphasis on orgasm.

Too much emphasis on orgasm? Orgasm a mistake? Orgasm a problem? In all my years of sex, I have heard orgasm called a lot of things—but a *problem*? Lack of orgasm— I have certainly heard that described as a problem, but could there really be such a thing as too much orgasm? Not at all! In fact, I think we should spend a whole lot more time focused on orgasm. Why? Because orgasm is a profoundly important physical and spiritual experience. Orgasm is the body's best natural therapy for relieving stress and tension; it is a naturally revitalizing and healing experience. Orgasm is our own personal little taste of the Great Cosmic Orgasm that connects us to All That Is. How could this possibly be a problem?

As a society, we've barely begun to explore orgasm, much less to understand how spiritually profound orgasm can be, and how many magical ways we can use it for our healing and happiness, and the health and happiness of others.

What Is Orgasm?

Which of the following do you think is the most accurate definition of orgasm?
  A. A sexual climax attained by stimulation of the genitals and other erogenous zones
  B. A release of accumulated tension and energy
  C. A release of tension and expansion of energy flowing through the body/mind and connecting us to spirit

Okay, it's a trick question—the correct answer is all of the above. But which kind of orgasm would you like to experience on a regular basis?

The purely physical, most limited definition of orgasm—answer A—has been our social and medical model. Orgasm is seldom observed outside the realm of sex and sexual activity, and then generally only within the realm of partner sex. Ninety-nine percent of the mass-market magazine articles on how to have a better orgasm are working within this definition. The most commonly experienced orgasm could be called the Mount St. Helen's orgasm. It's got a quick buildup and a rapid release, followed by a cooling down. The physical sensation is centered in your genitals and lower abdomen. It feels really good, though it's generally quite brief. After this kind of orgasm, you feel relaxed and possibly also sleepy. In all fairness to the misled sociologist on NPR, this may be the only kind of orgasm she has ever experienced. And that would be a problem.

Definition B, the kind of orgasm we experience when we suddenly release stored-up tension and energy, is in many ways similar to the Mount St. Helen's orgasm, with a major exception—it does not feel as localized. It is still a genital orgasm, but afterward you feel as though the tension has been drained out of your arms and legs. Your hands and fingers may tingle. Your chest feels more open, and you can breathe more easily and deeply. The relaxation is profound and satisfying. You may drop off to sleep. Better than orgasm type A—but wait, there's more!

The kind of orgasm that combines the release of tension and energy with the added plus of a spiritual connection to All That Is may (or may not) begin with the genitals. The orgasmic energy starts in the very center of your being, then flows out to the limits of your body and beyond. You may feel boundaryless, as if you can't tell where you end and everything else begins. You may feel as if you are in a sort of alternate universe where everything is beautiful, quiet, and peacefully connected. Your orgasm is happening everywhere and nowhere, and it may go on and on. Afterward you may feel energized, or you may feel peaceful and blissed-out. Anyone who has ever experienced this kind of orgasm would never label it problematic!

This kind of orgasm is not limited to sex, and it's certainly not limited to the genitals. When we expand our definition of orgasm, we are presented with a vast number of orgasmic experiences. Think about those unstoppable laugh attacks that take you over in waves of rolling silliness. They usually start with one funny line or sight gag, and roll on and on until everything and anything is funny and you're laughing so hard that your diaphragm is spasming and you're gasping for breath. It feels like you've lost all control of your laughter—the laugh is laughing you. How do you feel after one of these gigglegasms?

Now, remember a time you got angry—when you just lost it—a time when you let all your rage fly. The more anger you released, the more poured out. You screamed and swore and pounded and yelled so loudly that your throat was sore afterward. Remember how you felt after that angergasm?

How about tears? Can you remember a time when you started crying and couldn't stop? You sobbed so deeply that you thought you were going to cry your guts out. Do you remember how that crygasm felt? Was it healing? Good, even? Was it similar to how you felt after a gigglegasm? An angergasm?

Gigglegasms, angergasms, and crygasms all leave us feeling cleansed and energized. Emotiongasms are "total" experiences; you allow your body to express its emotions without trying to stifle them. This is how we behaved when we were young children, before we were socialized to behave more "acceptably." Emotiongasms are a liberation from tight bondage. In fact, as we try to "suck it up" and "tough our way through" life, our bodies produce bands of stress that leave us wrapped as tightly as a rubber band. In densely populated urban and suburban culture, we are especially prone to stuffing our emotions. There just isn't enough physical and psychic space to allow big, intense emotions without trespassing all over the psychic space of others.

Angergasms, crygasms, and gigglegasms may appear to be the spontaneous result of a powerful emotion we are feeling at the moment. But emotion is not the only source of an emotiongasm. Allow me to get technical for a moment, please.

The physiological ingredients of an emotiongasm are the same as a genital orgasm. A buildup of life force or sexual energy is brought about by a combination of breath, movement, sound, and muscular contractions and is followed by a release. This buildup and subsequent orgasmic release of life/sex energy doesn't necessarily depend on genital stimulation. Emotiongasms don't even depend on any particular emotion. In the course of a single breath and energy orgasm session (such as a Firebreath Orgasm or a Clench and Hold, which we will practice in chapter 9, "Breath and Energy Orgasms"), you could even have a gigglegasm, followed by a crygasm, followed by an angergasm, followed by another gigglegasm.

Not all energy orgasms are earth-shattering emotional catharses. Some of my favorite orgasms are tiny, fairy-like blissgasms. These are the little bites of bliss that start at your tailbone and wiggle their way up your spine until they explode like little sparklers in your brain. They usually happen when you are very quiet, perhaps just sitting looking out upon the ocean waves or at a sunset. But not always.

One particularly delightful blissgasm sneaked up on me one stunningly beautiful morning in Sydney, Australia. I was out for a stroll in the city, breathing in the clean, cool air, feeling the intense, hot sun on my skin, and being so grateful to be alive and in that beautiful city on that beautiful day. I've always subscribed to the theory that if you make love to the universe, the universe will make love to you, so I began using several of my favorite Tantric techniques to circulate sexual energy between me and Sydney. Nothing I was doing was obvious to anyone on the street; I'm sure I appeared to be nothing more than a smiling, happier-than-usual woman on her way to the post office. I had no big expectation of any particular climax as a result of my lovemaking with the city of Sydney. I most surely had no expectation of any particular physical sensation. But before I knew it, a little blissgasm shivered up my spine, followed by an actual clitoral orgasm that washed up the front of my body. These two waves crashed together in my head. I was so amazed, I had to stop and lean against a wall—I'd had a walking orgasm!

So, which was better, the blissgasm or the clitgasm? Is an energy orgasm better than a genital orgasm? No, they are simply different. But is an energy orgasm combined with a genital orgasm better than either one separately? You bet!

It may be hard to believe that a good cry or laugh can be an orgasm. It may be even harder to believe that you can have an orgasm simply walking down the street. But it is important that we accept these ecstatic states as a kind of orgasm. When we limit the possibilities of our orgasms, we limit our energy, which can limit all our possibilities.

But Wait, There's More!

All too often, women tell me that they have never had an orgasm. Understandably, they often have feelings of deep shame, grief, failure, and anger. Before we talk about how she might become orgasmic, I always ask a woman if she has experienced any gigglegasms, crygasms, or angergasms. Invariably she will say that she has, even if only as a child. There are no inorgasmic women; there are simply some women who have not yet experienced a genital orgasm. The moment an "inorgasmic" woman realizes that she is capable of orgasm—that she in fact has already had orgasms—she can open up to the possibilities of more, expanded genital orgasms.

I often ask workshop participants, "What would make your orgasms better?" The most popular answer is this: "I know there is something more out there and I would like to be able to let go and find it." I have heard this from both women and men (and from those creative beings who are somehow neither or both). People of vastly varied sexual experience all seem to know that there is something more. Whether your "something more" orgasm is a bigger, better physical orgasm, or you're longing for a rendezvous with your higher power, your desire for "something more" is your divinely legitimate right.

Before I move on to energetic techniques to expand your orgasmic possibilities, I want to give you some nuts-and-bolts tips on good old-fashioned physical orgasms. According to the principles of Taoism, yang energy builds quickly and dissipates quickly; yin energy builds slowly and dissipates slowly. Traditionally, it has been thought that men are more yang and women are more yin. However, today there are many transgender people who are neither one gender nor another. Yin and yang can no longer be assigned according to the shape of one's genitals. However, yin and yang can be closely aligned with the hormones that predominate in the body. People with testosterone-based bodies (whether they were born male or take testosterone as a supplement) tend to be more yang. People with estrogen-based bodies (whether they were born female or take estrogen as a supplement) are typically more yin.

The most common questions I hear from people on their way to those "something more" orgasms are these:

From people with estrogen-based bodies: How do I have an orgasm? How do I have an orgasm more easily?

From people with testosterone-based bodies: How can I delay orgasm? Can I really orgasm without ejaculating? And if I don't ejaculate, can I really have multiple orgasms?

Given the role of hormones, it makes perfect sense that people with estrogen-based bodies would want to heat up more quickly, and people with testosterone-based bodies might wish to cool down. Each of us is intuitively searching for balance. Whether you identify with (or your desires lean toward) the yin or the yang, when you strive for a balance of the two, you can create the orgasmic experience you desire.

For purposes of the following instruction only, I will presume that people with estrogen-based bodies have a vulva, clitoris, and vagina, and I will occasionally refer to them as women. I will also presume that people with testosterone-based bodies have a penis and testicles, and I will occasionally refer to them as men. I am well-aware that this is not the case for everyone. I trust that if you

Braingasms

Did you know that people who have no feeling at all below the waist—people with spinal cord injuries, for example—can still have orgasms? It's true. My friend Alison Partridge, a paraplegic sex therapist in Adelaide, Australia, has physical sensations only in her hands and arms, breasts (one has less feeling than the other), neck, and head. Yet, when her clitoris is stimulated, she can have an orgasm. Where does she feel her orgasm to be located? Well, sometimes she orgasms in her nipples, sometimes inside her head. She reports that there is a distinct difference between nipple orgasms and the ones inside her head, but that both are wonderful. She has even discovered that by changing positions during sex she can have multiple orgasms. Alison's experience illuminates the presence of numerous previously undiscovered neural pathways by which orgasmic energy can travel through the body to the brain. The more I study orgasm, the more convinced I am that orgasm "happens" primarily in the brain and that the intensely pleasurable feeling in our genitals—the kind that usually accompanies most of our orgasms—is only one of the many pleasures possible with orgasm.

are clever enough to create your own gender, you are certainly creative enough to adapt these tips for your own magnificently unique body.

Orgasm Tips for Estrogen-Based Bodies

The most effective I have for you is, *practice, practice, practice*. The best tip to find your orgasm is to look for it on a regular basis—by yourself. When you are alone, you can give yourself permission to take as long as you like and try anything you like. There is no one, surefire way to orgasm, but with practice and patience, you will develop a collection of techniques, toys, and fantasies that work for you. Here are some techniques to help you on your path.

Relax. Take a bath. Wrap your legs up around the faucet and let the water rush onto your clitoris. Or use a detachable shower head and adjust the spray to the most pleasurable pressure and speed. If you have access to a hot tub, position yourself over one of the jets.

Look and explore. Lie back and relax. Play some sexy music. Caress yourself all over; get into the mood. Use a mirror and your fingers to explore your vulva and clitoris. Find out where your sensitive spots are. Apply a water-based lube and try a variety of strokes. Concentrate primarily, but not entirely, on your clitoris.

Think sexy thoughts. Get creative and get explicit. Political correctness has no place here. Your fantasy may have a detailed plotline or may just be a series of erotic images. Challenge yourself to create something new and hotter than before. Or, watch an erotic video or read an erotic story.

Breathe and rock. As you breathe, rock your pelvis as though you are fucking (or being fucked by) someone. Don't hold your breath! No matter what, keep breathing. You may feel that you'll "lose" the orgasm when you breathe, but you won't; you'll just build up more and more sexual energy, which will create a better orgasm.

Vibrate. I have never understood how some women can tell me that they are desperate to have an orgasm, yet they don't want to use a vibrator. Good goddess, that's like saying you want to go to the moon but don't want to use a rocket to get there. Buy a vibrator! Using a vibrator will not desensitize your clitoris. If that were true, mine would be absolutely numb by now. If you use your vibrator for several minutes and then go back to using your fingers, you may not feel enough stimulation to bring yourself to orgasm with your fingers—but hey, that's not a problem unless the electricity fails. Of the many kinds of vibrators on the market, I prefer electric ones, particularly the Hitachi Magic Wand. Of the battery-operated types, my favorite is the Natural Contours line, developed by Candida Royalle (see the resources section at the end of the book).

Press, release, press, release. The key to orgasm for most people is a steady, repeated motion. However, varying the pressure on the clitoris is more effective than hard pressure alone. Pretend your clit is a doorbell: press, release, press, release. Try this with long, slow presses and releases, and then short, fast ones.

Add penetration. A dildo may dramatically increase your orgasmic ability by providing a feeling of fullness in the vagina and by stimulating your G-spot. For extra fun, place your vibrator on the end of the dildo.

If you get tired and nothing seems to be working, change your breathing or your fantasy, or take a short break. You'll shake off the numbness and feel a fresh surge of energy.

Continue the stimulation when you feel the beginnings of an orgasm. Lighten up during the first extremely sensitive moment, but keep the stimulation going to enjoy all the possible aftershocks.

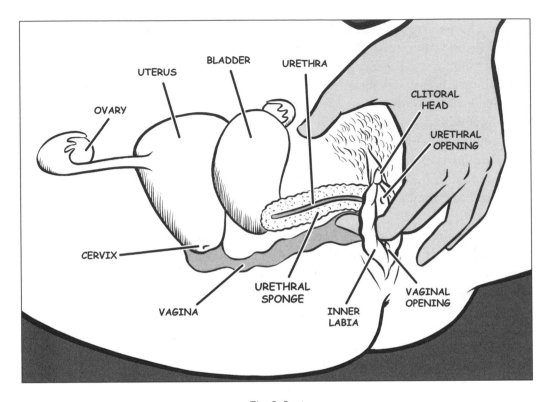

The G-Spot

WHAT ABOUT G-SPOT ORGASMS?

Is there such a thing as a G-spot orgasm? Sure there is. Women who enjoy G-spot orgasms describe them as feeling deeper and more diffuse than clitoral orgasms. The G-spot was named for Ernst Gräfenberg, the doctor credited with "discovering" this area on a woman's urethral sponge that, thousands of years before, had been named the Black Pearl by the Taoists.

The urethral sponge is the tissue that surrounds the urethra on the front wall of the vagina. Technically, the entire urethral sponge is the G-spot; however, many women do have a "spot" of erectile tissue (usually the size of a dime or a quarter, depending on the woman and how aroused she is) that has a slightly rougher—some might say ribbed—texture. The G-spot is most easily found by inserting a finger (palm up) into the vagina and making a "come here" gesture toward the front wall.

The tissue of the urethral sponge is actually an internal extension of the clitoris; however, there is a distinction between the two in that the sensations from the clitoris travel on the pudendal nerve, while sensations from the G-spot travel on the pelvic nerve, which also transmits sensations from the bladder. This would explain why stimulation of the G-spot often produces the feeling of needing to urinate.

Some women love having their G-spot stimulated; others feel it is too intense. Approach the G-spot gently. This area tends to hold any sexual trauma that a woman has experienced; intense feelings and even pain can be triggered if the G-spot is handled too roughly. Some women ejaculate when their G-spot is stimulated; others may ejaculate when their clitoris is stimulated. Many women do not ejaculate; although with practice, many can and do ejaculate copiously and blissfully.

Orgasm Tips for Testosterone-Based Bodies

Orgasm and ejaculation are two different physical processes. The Taoists knew this 3,000 years ago, but we in the West are only now beginning to acknowledge the difference. Those clever Taoists discovered that if you can delay or withhold your ejaculation, you can experience multiple orgasms. In addition, according to Taoist sexuality (which began as a branch of Chinese medicine), men can live longer and increase their vitality by avoiding the exhaustion and loss of energy that follow ejaculation. According to the Tao, the body will use the energy it saves by not having to replenish sperm to nourish the mind, body, and spirit.

Most men equate orgasm with ejaculation, so it can be difficult to imagine the two separated. Ejaculation is simply a reflex, a muscle spasm triggered by orgasm. Orgasm happens just before ejaculation. In fact, men are capable of multiple orgasms. And why shouldn't they be? I've done years of work with men, women, and those who are something else entirely, and I am more and more convinced that "male" and "female" genitals and sexuality are a lot more alike than they are different.

The truth is, men are not from Mars and women are not from Venus. We are all earthlings whose penises and vaginas came from exactly the same type of fetal tissue. This is why, in addition to penises and vaginas, we also have a wide spectrum of intersex genitals, which medical science is only now slowly coming to accept as "normal."

TEN WAYS TO DELAY EJACULATION

Practice these techniques alone, at first. Then you can share them with a partner who can help you. Give yourself at least twenty minutes. Masturbate almost to the point of orgasm. As you approach orgasm, notice what is happening in your body. What muscles are you tensing? How are you breathing? What are you doing that is speeding up ejaculation? Now, just as you are on the verge of orgasm:

1. Stop stroking or thrusting your penis for ten to twenty seconds. Go totally limp, completely soft inside. During this moment of relaxation, take your focus off your genitals. Direct it to the top of your head or your third eye. You'll feel your orgasmic energy remain in motion, even though the muscles of your genitals are not.

2. Breathe in and hold your breath for several moments, until the urge to ejaculate subsides. Remember, the more you breathe, the more you feel. In this case, you want to decrease sensation. If this doesn't work, try a fast, shallow breath like the Breath of Fire (see chapter 4).

3. Contract and hold the PC muscle. This is similar to a Kegel exercise (see chapter 7). You'll have to practice to find exactly the right timing for this. The PC muscle surrounds your prostate. By learning to squeeze your prostate while it is contracting involuntarily, you can stop ejaculation just before the point of no return.

4. Find your perineum—the area between your anus and your testicles. While contracting your PC muscle, press a finger into this point, up to your first knuckle. This may sound strange, but it works.

5. Place two fingers on the underside of your penis, place your thumb on top, and squeeze.

6. Holding your penis in one hand, press down on the tip with your thumb.

7. Holding your penis between two fingers and your thumb, squeeze at the base.

8. Lie on your back. Gravity will draw blood away from your erection. (If you are already on your back, lift your hips.)

9. Pull your scrotal sac down and away from your body. (Your testicles pull up close to the body when you are about to ejaculate.)

10. Relaxation is the key to voluntary ejaculation. This is easier to learn in passive, receptive mode; so when you're with your lover, lie back and let her/him get on top. Let your lover be the surfer and you the surfboard. Relax, breathe, and slow down.

Remember, sexual energy will flow wherever you put your attention. If you keep all your focus on your groin—even if you are focusing on stopping your penis from ejaculating—this is where the energy will flow, and you will ejaculate. When you focus on circulating sexual energy throughout your entire body, you will be able to enjoy orgasmic feelings in other parts of your body, such as your chest, belly, or head. You may even have whole-body orgasms.

What about P-Spot Orgasms?

The prostate gland is located behind the pubic bone and just below the bladder, near the internal root of the penis. The prostate corresponds to the G-spot in women and, like the G-spot, is connected to the pelvic nerve rather than the pudendal nerve. The P-spot is particularly well situated to produce deep, intensely pleasurable sensations, including orgasm.

You cannot massage the P-spot directly. It can only be accessed through the anus, which is filled with millions of delicately sensitive nerve endings. (In postoperative transgender women, the prostate can also be accessed through the back wall of the surgically constructed vagina.) The prostate itself is highly sensitive to pressure. Pressing, rubbing, or stroking the gland through the rectal wall can produce sublime and profound orgasms, especially if the receiver is highly aroused.

You can massage the prostate by inserting a gloved, lubed finger two to three inches into the rectum and stroking toward the front of the body. Gloves are recommended in order to protect the delicate anal membranes from sharp fingernails and rough skin. You can also use a dildo or an insertable vibrator, although a finger is the best way to find the prostate. You'll feel it as a walnut-sized bulge, although it may be larger in men over forty. As with the G-spot, a man might find P-spot massage irritating if he is not already aroused. And, also like the G-spot, the P-spot can hold strong emotional feelings. Start slowly and let the receiver set the pace.

Whatever your favorite path to orgasm, please remember: there is no right way or wrong way to have an orgasm. Orgasms vary in intensity, duration, and location, but there is simply no such thing as a bad orgasm! As you practice Tantra, you'll be practicing new ways of moving sexual energy through your body. And as you do, you will probably discover new and expanded varieties of orgasms.

Orgasmic Sounds

One surefire way to have bigger, better, more intense orgasms is to open up your throat chakra and make some noise. Have you ever seen Meg Ryan's luncheonette demonstration of how to fake an orgasm in the film *When Harry Met Sally*? She puts down her sandwich and begins to moan, starting with a low *ooo*, and then a slightly higher *ohh*. As she gets more and more "turned on," the pitch of her voice rises. "*Ahh*, yes, *ahh*, yes," she begs. At the peak of her faux orgasm, she lets go with a high-pitched "YES-SSSSS!!!!!" It's quite a good example of how erotic energy flows up the body on waves of sound.

In addition to pitch, each chakra has a corresponding syllable (or syllables, depending on the yogic tradition you follow). For building erotic energy, I have found these to be the most effective:

* First and second (root and sex) chakras: a very low *ooo* (as in *goose*)
* Third (solar plexus) chakra: a somewhat higher pitched *ohh* (as in *open*)
* Fourth (heart) chakra: a somewhat higher pitched *ahh* (as in *art*)
* Fifth (throat) chakra: a somewhat higher pitch *aay* (as in *play*)
* Sixth and seventh (third eye and crown) chakras: a very high pitched *eee* (as in *peep*)

Where's That Orgasm?

Funny but true: If you have sexually expressive neighbors, thin walls, and a taste for voyeurism, you'll have a fun time playing "Where's that orgasm?" You can tell where someone's sexual energy is by paying attention to the pitch of the sounds they're making. For instance, Meg Ryan seemed to be having an orgasm somewhere between a heartgasm and a throatgasm.

Knowing how to locate orgasmic energy, besides being a fun parlor game, is very useful when you're with a partner. If your partner is making very low sounds, you could play with their nipples, gently kiss their neck, or vibrate the top of their head to coax the energy upward. If your partner isn't making any kind of sound, encourage them to do so!

These sounds energize your body and start your chakras spinning. I often do the following exercise at the end of a busy work day to give me the energy to enjoy a fun evening. You can do this alone or facing a partner.

✳

Chakra Sounds

1. Sit or stand comfortably and keep your spine straight.
2. Start with a very low *ooo*. Feel the sound vibrate deep in your genitals and lower abdomen.
3. Raise the pitch a little and let *ohh* vibrate your solar plexus. Stay with it. Change pitches slightly until you can actually feel the vibration in your solar plexus.
4. Sing or chant a somewhat higher-pitched *ahh*. Let your shoulders relax and feel your chest expand. You'll know it's the right pitch when you feel the maximum vibration or expansion around your heart.
5. Next, sing or chant *aay*. Make sure you've raised the pitch from the previous chakra. Keep adjusting the pitch until you find the one that gives you the best vibration in your throat.
6. Last, sing or chant *eee* at the highest pitch you can comfortably reach. Let it vibrate the top of your head!

Energy will follow sound. You are moving sexual energy up your body with each higher-pitched sound you make. If you feel too much energy accumulating around your head, then make lower, more guttural sounds to pull it back down. I like to alternate between genital (first chakra), heart (fourth chakra), and third eye (sixth chakra) sounds. Not only do the sounds build and distribute sexual energy, they also release tension or pent-up emotions that might prevent the energy from moving freely through those chakras.

The Universal Hum

As an experiment, my friend Annie Sprinkle and I decided to see if we could have an orgasm by simply making sounds. We sat facing each other in a nice warm bath and began making sexy sounds as we gazed into each other's eyes. We warmed up with low, grunty sounds, moved on to breathy, throaty sounds, and then moved to high-pitched, "oh-my-god-I'm-coming" sounds. We faked it until we felt it. As my sexual energy started to build, I became less aware of the sounds I was making and more aware of what I was hearing. At first, of course, I heard the sounds Annie was making and the splashing of the bathwater. Then those sounds faded into the background, and I was acutely aware of honking taxicabs and other city street sounds. This was odd, since I was usually unaware of those sounds while in Annie's apartment, fourteen floors up from the street. All the apartment windows were closed, yet it was as if I were surrounded by a city full of sounds. I was no longer "doing" sounds, sounds were "doing" me. I floated into some vast space that certainly wasn't Annie's apartment. I heard the beginning of a hum. It was deeply soothing and comforting and drew me toward it. The hum grew louder and louder until it filled me inside and out. It was bliss. It wasn't until years later that I read that Annie and I had stumbled onto what yogis and mystics call the Universal Hum.

I have no idea how long I stayed inside the hum. I know I happily could have stayed there forever, but eventually I started to come back to Annie and the bathtub. We were totally blissed. Had we achieved our goal of using sounds to have an orgasm? We called it a blissgasm. Whatever it was, it was mind-blowing.

Once our understanding and awareness of something has expanded, it stays expanded. We can't shrink our consciousness by unthinking the thoughts that caused it to grow. Now that you are aware of the totality of possibilities of orgasm, there is no going back to your old, more limited view. So let's keep going. Dive with me into the next chapter of infinite ecstatic possibilities: breath and energy orgasms.

CHAPTER 9

Breath and Energy Orgasms

When I decided I wanted to wear a permanent symbol of my commitment to my Tantric path, I knew I had to go to my friend Pat. When Pat Sinatra tattoos you, it's an erotic healing experience. The tattoo we created was a woman standing on a coiled cobra holding a thousand-petaled lotus. Despite Pat's advice that tattooing over bone was some fresh new kind of hell, I resisted all her attempts to place the tattoo on the muscle above my ankle bone. I insisted it had to go directly on my ankle. Pat began inking the tattoo. She was right. Tattooing over bone was a bitch. As she did all the fine-needled black work—the outline and the bottom of the snake—I tried to find a way to breathe to help me cope with the pain. Pat works fast, and before long, I'd found a breath and she'd finished the outline. Now for the colors—Pat worked in one color ink at a time, and we agreed that I would breathe in the meaning of the chakra that corresponded to whatever color she'd be using. We began with red, the root chakra. It was right on the ankle bone and it felt like hammered fire. I began breathing a variation of the Circular Breath I regularly used to circulate sexual energy. Gradually, the pain started to go away! I started feeling quite floaty and I began to giggle. The giggle became a laugh. A huge ball of energy rolled up my leg, up my abdomen, and burst out of my heart in an explosion of joy. It was a spontaneous release of all the tension that had been accumulating in my ankle. "*Okay*, that's the first chakra," Pat said, finishing the red.

"Was it good for you?' I giggled. "That was amazing. I wonder if I can do that again?"

"Let's try," she grinned. "Here comes orange for the second chakra."

I kept breathing. To my astonishment, every chakra color Pat tattooed produced another energy orgasm. Some of them felt like they were centered in the chakra we were focusing on; others did not. Some were quiet; some were screamgasms. They were all fabulous! Other people enjoyed them, too. When another tattoo artist finished with her client, the two of them joined us, playing music and breathing with me. It was one totally incredible ritual and one miraculous afternoon. I was stoned on the energy until late that night when I fell into a most blissfully peaceful sleep.

95

What's So Special about Breath and Energy Orgasms?

As a child, my biggest thrill was doing whatever it was that people said I could not do. If someone told me that I couldn't take my bicycle apart and put it back together again, I'd have it in pieces in the driveway within the next hour and back together again by lunchtime. So, when someone told me it's not possible to have a real orgasm just by breathing, I wanted to prove otherwise. Never has proving something been so enjoyable! I simply adore breath and energy orgasms. They have given me hours of profound healing and insight, as well as some of the most fun I've ever had. They give me gigglegasms, angergasms, crygasms, and blissgasms. They clean out old emotional gunk and make me feel rested and new. They make me feel centered, expansive, and powerful. I have used them to stop smoking, to heal the pain of loss, to grieve the deaths of loved ones, and to visualize new career paths. I have breathed my way to orgasm as physical prayer, and as a group alternative to a round of martinis at a boring cocktail party. I have done breath and energy orgasms alone, with partners, and in groups. The possibilities are endless.

The Firebreath Orgasm

Although its name is similar to the Breath of Fire, the Firebreath Orgasm is a completely different breath process. The Firebreath Orgasm was so named by Harley Swiftdeer, Cherokee medicine man, activist, and teacher; but variations of this technique are found in all sexually knowledgeable and sex-positive cultures of the past, such as the Tantrists and Taoists, as well as in the modern therapy work of Wilhelm Reich and Alexander Lowen. This technique can be a deeply healing and enlightening sexual meditation, producing waves of tingly sexual pleasure that surge through every part of the body. You may experience profound relaxation and powerful insights about your life or life in general. You may feel reborn. You will almost certainly discover a deeply meaningful thread running through breath, emotion, energy, and pleasure.

BEFORE YOU BEGIN

Here are some pointers to keep in mind before you attempt the Firebreath Orgasm.

* You may want to practice with a friend who can read the instructions to you; or, you can read the instructions into a tape recorder and play them back.
* The Firebreath Orgasm can be done as a conscious quickie in about twenty minutes. However, the first few times you try it, you may want to allow more time.
* Drop your expectations—the good ones and the bad ones. If you are thinking that this will never work for you, or that it will be the most profound experience you've ever had, you're setting yourself up for disappointment. Keep your mind focused on your breath and on what you are feeling in the present moment, not what could happen in the future.
* People respond differently to breath and energy orgasm techniques, and it may take a while for you to feel the "orgasm" part. For example, I was swept away in waves of pleasure the first time I did the Firebreath Orgasm, but it took months of practice to feel the bliss of another technique, called the Clench and Hold (discussed later in this chapter). My friend Annie's experience was exactly the reverse. Be patient with yourself.
* The Firebreath Orgasm is a powerful process. It can produce feelings of great intensity, including feelings of anger or sadness. This is completely normal. If it happens, just keep breathing through any unpleasant feelings that come up. These are not feelings you have to sit in and process for months before you get to the pleasure. They are simply emotions that come up to be cleared out. Allow them, but do not get lost in them. Keep your intention on pleasure. Think of the negative feelings as small clouds in an endless blue sky of pleasure, and simply watch them pass by.
* You may feel a pleasant tingling sensation in your hands, face, or feet. This yummy tingling may spread throughout your whole body. Occasionally, the tingling may intensify into a tight, cramping feeling, typically in your hands or lips. This is not dangerous, although it can feel a bit weird. Slow your breathing down and try to relax. The cramping will pass. The cramping appears to be the result of stress or tension in combination with the presence of increased oxygen in the body. I think of it as the conflict that results when the body tries to hang on to tension at the same time the breath tries to release it. The more breath work you do, the less likely you'll experience cramping.

* The Firebreath Orgasm is a chakra-oriented meditation. You will be breathing into each chakra. As you do so, you may want to meditate on the color or affirmations appropriate to each chakra. This can be very healing and will help you keep your focus.
* You'll be breathing energy up your body in circles. When the energy reaches your upper chakras, it will start to do you instead of you doing it. Simply enjoy it, and *keep breathing*!
* I'm going to show you two ways to do the Firebreath Orgasm. Many people find the simplified version just as effective as the full version, and easier to do. I suggest you read both before trying either. Then try the version that seems the most appropriate for you.

The Firebreath Orgasm: The Full Version

1. Lie comfortably on your back, with your knees up and your feet flat on the floor. Keep your spine straight. Don't use a pillow.
2. Relax your jaw. Yawn. Keep the back of your throat open.
3. Breathe in through your nose and exhale through your mouth. If you're not comfortable breathing in through your nose, feel free to breathe in and out through your mouth. The important thing is to take in as much air as possible in a relaxed manner.
4. Think of your breath as a circle, with no pause between the inhale and the exhale. Don't force the exhale.
5. As you inhale, let your belly fill up like a balloon. As you exhale, flatten your lower back to the ground. This rocking motion helps to move sexual energy.
6. Add Kegels (see chapter 7). Most people like to squeeze on the exhale, but do what feels right for you.
7. Now, use your mind and your breath to pull energy into your perineum (the area between your genitals and your anus—a.k.a. the root chakra). Remember, energy easily follows thought. You do not have to push and pull the energy; all you have to do is focus on the chakra you are breathing into, and the breath will follow. You may find it helpful to place your hands on the chakra into which you are breathing.
8. Now, inhale your energy up to the sex center (lower belly, at the second chakra).

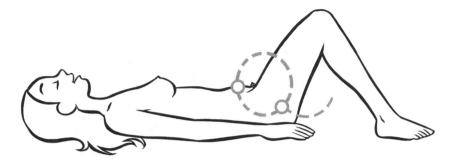

First chakra to second chakra

9. Exhale, circulating the energy back down to the perineum. Continue until your sex center feels charged up, lit up, bigger, or more alive. Trust yourself; you'll know when it is charged. You will feel that you're ready to move on, or as if the energy is moving up by itself.

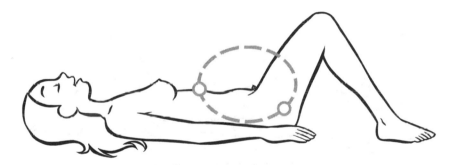

First chakra to third chakra

10. Now enlarge the circle. Breathe energy between your perineum (first chakra) and your solar plexus (third chakra). It's located below your diaphragm and above your belly button. Keep rocking and Kegeling. Continue until this area is well charged up.

11. Now reduce the circle, circulating energy from your sex center (second chakra) to solar plexus center (third chakra).

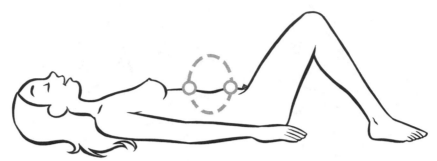

Second chakra to third chakra

12. Keep breathing! By now you may (or may not) be feeling some of the physical or emotional effects of the Firebreath Orgasm.
13. Enlarge the circle so that you are breathing the energy between your sex center (second chakra) and your heart (fourth chakra). When that feels complete, reduce the circle so that energy is circulating between your solar plexus (third chakra) and heart center (fourth chakra).

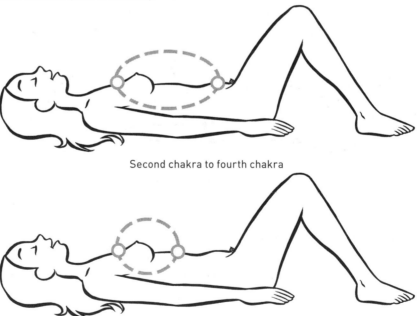

Second chakra to fourth chakra

Third chakra to fourth chakra

14. Are you seeing the pattern here? The next circle is from your solar plexus (third chakra) to your throat (fifth chakra), followed by a smaller circle between your heart (fourth chakra) and your throat (fifth chakra). By the time the energy reaches your throat, you'll probably want to make some sounds. If sighs or sounds haven't happened naturally yet, it's important to vocalize them at this point. It will help the energy move up.

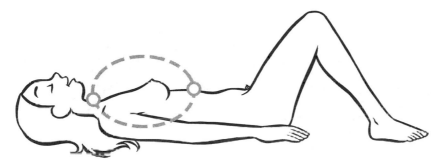

Third chakra to fifth chakra

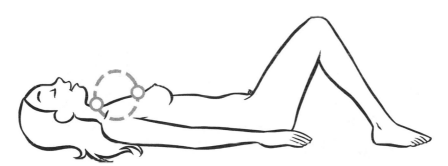

Fourth chakra to fifth chakra

15. By now, the energy may or may not be moving up the chakras on its own. If it is, just keep breathing the connected breath; you can stop visualizing the circles. If the energy is not yet moving on its own, your next circle is from the heart (fourth chakra) to the third eye (the middle of your forehead—the sixth chakra), followed by a smaller circle between the throat (fifth chakra) and third eye (sixth chakra). Roll your eyes up (while closed) as though you can see out the top of your head; it will help the energy rise.

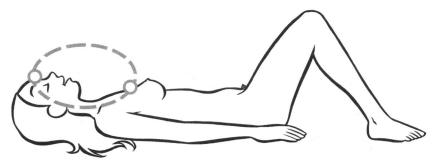

Fourth chakra to sixth chakra

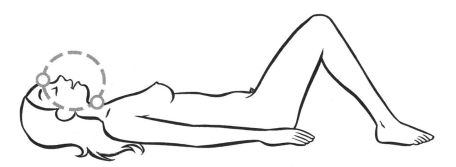

Fifth chakra to sixth chakra

16. The next circle is from the throat (fifth chakra) to the crown (just above the top of your head—the seventh chakra), followed by the smaller circle between the third eye (sixth chakra) and the crown (seventh chakra).

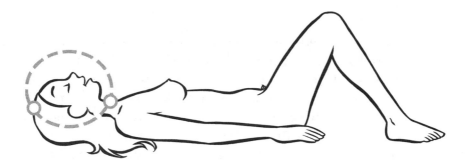

Fifth chakra to seventh chakra

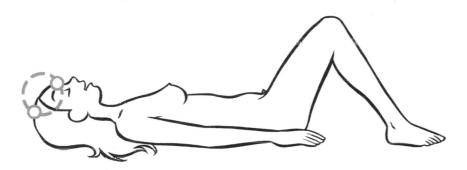

Sixth chakra to seventh chakra

Remember, by the time you reach these higher circles, the energy will most likely be flowing on its own. Just keep breathing and you will feel yourself moving rapidly into an orgasmic state.

HELPFUL HINTS

If at any point in the process you feel that you have lost the plot and aren't feeling anything, don't get discouraged, and don't think you're doing something wrong. Energy levels may rise and fall. Just return to the level where the energy seems to have settled, and start again from there. Or, go all the way back to the root chakra and pull energy from there directly into whichever higher chakra you're trying to energize.

Stay focused on your breath circles by using your hands to touch the chakras you're breathing into. Or, move your hands in small circles, as if lifting the energy up with each inhalation.

Raise the pitch of your voice on your exhalations as you move the energy up each chakra. This is particularly true as you circle energy in the higher chakras.

Remember, do not be alarmed if you experience lightheadedness; dizziness; or tingling sensations, spasms, or constrictions in your hands and feet. These effects are only temporary. Take slow, deep breaths. The symptoms should pass in a short time. If you experience these symptoms, it may mean you are trying too hard. Ease up!

※
The Firebreath Orgasm: The Simplified Version

The simplified version is exactly the same as the full version, except in the sequence of the chakras through which you circle energy up your body. Instead of circulating energy between chakras one and two, then one and three, then two and three, then two and four, then three and four, and so on, you simply circulate the energy as follows:

Between the perineum and sex center *(first and second chakras)*

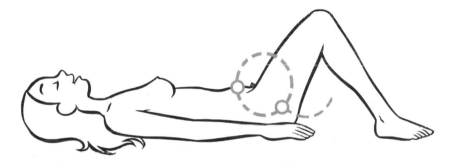

Between the sex center and solar plexus *(second and third chakras)*

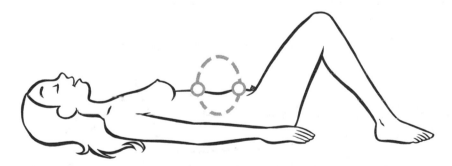

Between the solar plexus and heart *(third and fourth chakras)*

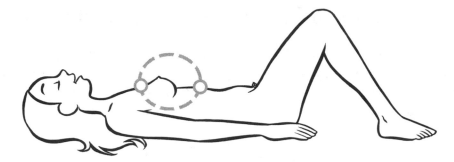

Between the heart and throat *(fourth and fifth chakras)*

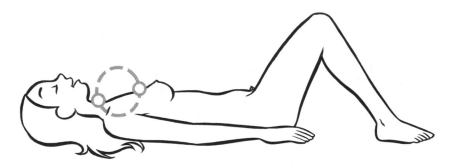

Between the throat and the third eye *(fifth and sixth chakras)*

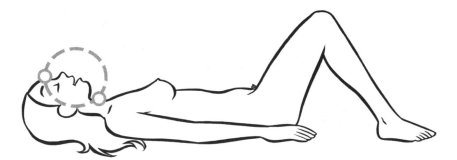

Between the third eye and the crown *(sixth and seventh chakras)*

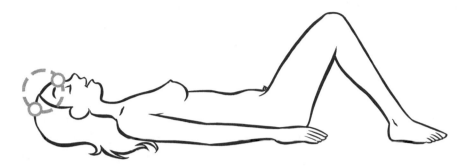

Energize each chakra as you go. Everything else is the same.

ARE YOU BREATHING?

Is reading these long descriptions of breath techniques making your brain bleed? If so, this would be a great time to practice one of the four conscious breaths outlined in chapter 4. Pick one, and breathe until you're back in your body. Then, if you have twenty to sixty minutes, take the phone off the hook and try the Firebreath Orgasm.

The Clench and Hold

The Clench and Hold is a Taoist technique I first learned from Joseph Kramer at his Friday evening "Breathe and Dance until You Come" parties (he called them Tantric Group Rebirths) in New York in the late 1980s. It took a lot of practice for me to feel the power of this process, and it was worth it. The Clench and Hold is my favorite breath orgasm technique. I like to practice it not only as an exercise by itself but also with partners and while having sex. I have explored numerous variations of it, but its essence remains the same.

The way the Clench and Hold works is quite simple: you breathe. Your body relaxes and becomes charged with energy. Then you constrict most of the muscles in your body. Finally, you let go and do nothing. What happens? You never know. You may have a catharsis, or you may see visions. You may tingle all over, or you may feel deeply quiet and peaceful. You may have insights, or you may feel as if you are making love to some form of deity. You may feel as if you have achieved an ecstatic death.

Why the Clench and Hold works is open to interpretation. The Taoist opinion is that when you build lots of energy through breath and movement and then suddenly stop and constrict your muscles, there is nowhere for all that energy to go but up through your central energy channel (the Inner Flute) and out the top of your head (in a process known as the Ejection of Consciousness)—hence, the feeling of blasting off that many people experience. However, I think of the blast-off as more of a blast *inward* or an *injection* of consciousness.

For years, I subscribed to the notion that there was something more spiritually "pure" about the upper chakras, and I tried endlessly to blast out of my body into some higher, more esoteric realm. Once, as I was enjoying the afterglow of a particularly powerful Clench and Hold, I felt myself blasting inward. I realized that true higher wisdom was inside me, not out in some other realm. It was a vacuum drawing insight inward—an *injection* of consciousness.

❊

The Clench and Hold

Before you actually start this breath orgasm, please read through the instructions and then rehearse the individual steps to help your body learn the process.

First, we'll charge the body with breath.

1. Sit comfortably on the floor.
2. Relax your jaw.
3. Yawn. Keep the back of your throat open.
4. Breathe using the Heart Breath (see chapter 4). Breathe in through your mouth using as little effort as possible. Take in as much air as you can with the least possible effort.
5. Let go. Let the exhale simply fall out. Let it fall out with a sigh. This relaxed little sound will show that you aren't pushing the breath out.
6. Keep your eyes open. Focus on a point somewhere in the room. You want to stay conscious with your breath and not nod off.
7. Keep breathing. If you want, you can gently rock back and forth with the breath. You can add Kegels. Make it erotic. Let it feel good. Just remember to stay with the breath.
8. Set a timer. Breathe for ten minutes—or twenty or thirty! The more you breathe, the more you charge up the body.

9. When you're ready to do the Clench and Hold, take thirty or so fuller, faster breaths to really charge up.

10. Lie back on the floor.

11. Take a full, deep breath. Fill up your lungs from bottom to top. Then let it all go without forcing your breath out.

12. Take another full, deep breath, and let it go, gently and fully.

13. Take a third deep breath. Fill up with as much air as you can hold . . . and . . . hold that breath!

14. Now here's the important part: as you're holding in your third deep breath, clench every muscle in your body, especially your abdominal muscles, your butt muscles, and your PC muscle. It won't matter much if your hands or your feet aren't clenched, but if your abs, butt, and PC muscle aren't clenched, the Clench and Hold won't be as effective.

    There are a number of ways to do this clench.

    Lying on your back, you'll want to make sure that you don't put undue stress on your neck or lower back when you tense up, so take a moment and rehearse how you are going to clench before you start breathing. One good way to create the tension you're looking for is to press down into the floor. Try it.

    Press down into the floor with your hands, shoulders, head, butt, legs, and feet.

    Alternatively, extend your body as far as it can go, and reach for opposite walls with your feet and hands.

    Or, pull in toward the center of your body as hard as you can—first clench your abs, and then pull the rest of your body in toward your abs.

    However you do it, make sure you don't bring your knees up toward your stomach. This releases your abdominal muscles, and that's exactly what you don't want to do!

15. Keep clenching for about fifteen seconds, and then let go.

16. Now, here's the hardest part of the Clench and Hold for most people: have no expectations. Don't try to make anything happen. You have given yourself a huge gift of openness and energy. Just be.

Breath and energy orgasms are mind-blowing in every sense of the word. They shatter our preconceived notions of how sex, pleasure, and bodies work. This is a good thing. Nothing remarkable was ever discovered without a mind or two being blown. Breath and energy orgasms may seem magical to you, but once you accept that one can (or has) happened to you, all sorts of other "magical" moments may reveal themselves—not only sexually, but in other areas of your life as well. Use your capacity for magical thinking: what else might my body be capable of doing that I hadn't considered? How many other sexual/spiritual possibilities might be out there waiting to delight me? Read on. In the next chapter, you'll see how solo Tantra is a perfect way to discover these new possibilities.

CHAPTER 10

Solo Tantra

Most of us live in or grew up in a culture that places a heavy emphasis on the importance of monogamous coupledom. The romantic myth, in all its impossible glory, remains the model relationship most of us have sought at one time or another. We looked for that one knight in shining armor (or damsel in distress) to sweep us off our feet, meet all our physical and emotional needs, and fuck us into the bliss of our dreams for the rest of our lives. We may know intellectually or even logically that this mythical notion of romantic pairing is impossible to achieve; yet we still think of it as the model for the ideal relationship. So we try to come as close to achieving it as we can.

If you are a longtime subscriber to the romantic myth, you may have a hard time believing that there is any value or fun in solo Tantra. You may be preoccupied with the thought that you still haven't found anyone with whom to practice real Tantra (that is, Tantra with a partner). Even if you have a sexual partner (or several), solo Tantra will introduce you to new aspects of your sexuality. It will give you the time and space to practice focusing on your own sexual energy and desires.

I have always loved solo Tantra. I have used it to discover and fall in love with myself. I have used it as creative inspiration, sexual meditation, sexual prayer, and a way of getting in touch with myself before connecting with others. For me, the essence of solo Tantra is the heart-genital connection. When I was first exploring solo Tantra, I ran across a simple exercise in a wonderful little book called *Masturbation, Tantra and Self Love*, by Margo Woods. With one hand, I masturbated using a vibrator (or my hand, dildo, or whatever). I placed the other hand on my heart. Just before I was about to orgasm, I stopped masturbating and breathed the orgasmic energy into my heart. I did this two more times before I finally let myself orgasm. I still practice this technique regularly. A wave of sexual energy rolls into my heart, flooding it with love and compassion.

Bringing sexual energy up to the heart can be effective and rewarding in a variety of situations, and it can produce some unexpectedly profound experiences.

My friend and favorite piercer, Raelyn Gallina, is someone I've always been able to count on for a piercing with serious spiritual content. On one of her annual visits to New York from her home in San Francisco, I scheduled an appointment for a piercing.

I decided on a clit hood piercing ritual that would deepen the connection between my heart and my clit.

I sat on a chair with my knees apart and my feet flat on the floor. I grounded myself like a tree with huge long roots that reached all the way into the center of the earth. "Say 'Now' when you're ready," Raelyn said. I was doing the Heart Breath and focusing all my attention on my heart chakra. "Now," I said. Suddenly, a huge, hot ball of energy shot up the front of my body, exploded out of my heart, and melted as it flooded down my chest and arms. Then a huge, white-violet firecracker of energy burst in slow motion on top of and in front of my head. I had no awareness of my clit, but every other part of my body was tingling. My mind suddenly expanded; it felt as though all the molecules in my body and mind had taken three giant steps away from each other. I was a permeable membrane through which everything and everyone could pass. I felt love for and connection with everything. I was going through an overwhelmingly beautiful expression of the highest heart energy: compassion for all beings.

That's what the right genital piercings performed by the right piercer at the right time can do. However, if genital piercings do not appeal to you as a tool for sexual, spiritual, and emotional advancement, that's fine. What meditations or practices might you use to connect your sexuality with your heart?

Eye Gazing

It is said with good reason that the eyes are the gateway to the soul. In Tantra, we spend a lot of time gazing into the eyes of another person. This can be challenging. Eye gazing takes us to a level of intimacy we experience infrequently; it tends to make us very uncomfortable. We may feel exposed, put on the spot, and even silly. We may feel the urge to look away, or we might start to giggle. Eye gazing is a trust exercise of the highest order. Regular practice of this exercise will make eye gazing easier.

❉

Gazing into Your Own Eyes

1. Hold a hand mirror in one hand, and place your other hand on your heart.
2. Look into the mirror, and look into your own nondominant eye. (If you are right-handed, your left eye is your nondominant eye; if you are left-handed, it's your right eye.)

3. Breathe.
4. As you gaze into your own eye, have an intimate dialogue with yourself. Try to speak it out loud. If that makes you feel too uncomfortable, say it silently. As you become more comfortable with this kind of intimacy, it will become easier to speak. Try using the following as a guideline for your dialogue. Just complete these statements with as much truth and love as you can.

   > I love you for . . .
   > I forgive you for . . .
   > If I really loved you, I would . . .
   > Because I really love you, I will . . .

If this sounds too New-Agey to be true, I empathize. I once thought that way. But I realized that if I couldn't have this simple dialogue with myself, I was kidding myself into thinking I could have real intimacy with someone else. Intimacy had always been a dangerous game for me. As I was growing up, I couldn't be open and honest with my parents. When I did try to be clear and truthful about who I was, what I did, and what I thought or felt, I was either punished or yelled at. I'd learned that being intimate with someone was the equivalent of shooting myself in the foot. It took me a long time and a lot of work to open up and trust the people I love and who love me. Mirror work like this eye gazing exercise was one of my most powerful tools in that process.

Intimacy is love expressed with trust, courage, attentiveness, and honesty. I'll bet you can find at least one of these qualities inside yourself—perhaps all four. Dive right in. Practice open-eyed orgasms. Masturbate while looking into a mirror and look into your own eyes as you orgasm. As you come, tell yourself how sexy you are and how much you love yourself.

The Microcosmic Orbit

The primary bioelectric circuit along which life/sex energy runs in your body is called the Microcosmic Orbit. Blockages to the free flow of life/sex energy accumulate along the Microcosmic Orbit as a result of the pressures and strains of modern life, such as stressful work, poor diet, shallow breathing, poor posture, and lack of exercise. Blocked energy can be manifested as fatigue, illness, and a weak immune system. When you consciously circulate energy around the Microcosmic Orbit, you begin to clear these blockages, and you can enjoy a sexier, more energized, and ecstatic life.

❄

The Microcosmic Orbit

1. Stand or sit comfortably with your feet flat on the floor and your spine straight.
2. Place your awareness at your perineum. Breathe in, drawing energy up and around to your tailbone. Then draw that energy up through your spine and neck, over the top of your head, and finally down your forehead to the roof of your mouth.
3. Place the tip of your tongue on the roof of your mouth. This connects the back and front channels.
4. Exhale, letting the energy trickle down the front of your body, over your genitals, and back to your perineum.
5. Repeat. This time, make it sexier. As you inhale, use a Kegel or two to pump the energy up your spine. Imagine that you are wrapping yourself in an egg-shaped cocoon of your own erotic energy. Feel that egg of energy. Give it a color, a texture, a sound, a smell, and a taste.

With regular practice, the Microcosmic Orbit will enter into your muscle memory and you won't have to think so hard to keep the orbit going. Then you can add masturbation. Practice circulating your own erotic energy until it becomes as natural, easy, and common as breathing.

Vibrate Those Chakras

This is a simple and effective way to wake up all your chakras and energize your entire body. I learned this from Betty Dodson, in her Bodysex workshop.

Starting at the first chakra, hold an electric vibrator to your body at all seven chakra points: the perineum, the sex center (lower abdomen), the solar plexus, the heart, the throat, the third eye (forehead), and the crown (top of the head). When you are vibrating over bone or a sensitive area—that is, the four upper chakras—place your hand between the vibrator and your body to make the vibration less intense. When you get to the top of your head, vibrate your way back down again if you like.

Masturbation is a great activity to accompany a chakra meditation. As you vibrate your chakras, notice which chakras are more (or less) sensitive than the rest. You can masturbate with the intention of soothing or bringing healing to these chakras. You can also dedicate or send your orgasm to that chakra and, in the afterglow, ask if there is something you need to know from that chakra to bring your body, emotions, or life into balance.

Discover What Truly Turns You On

Which of the following would be most likely to turn you on?

* Watching a lover do a tantalizing striptease
* Hearing a lover say sexy things to you
* Being stroked seductively

If you picked watching the striptease, you are most likely a visual person. If you chose having sexy little somethings whispered into your ear, you are probably auditory. And if being stroked slowly and seductively does it for you, you are most likely kinesthetic.

Each of us has a sense through which we prefer to take in and process the information we receive from the world around us. Some people process information in pictures and images, others in sounds. Still others perceive sensuality chiefly through physical sensations. For example, if three people with different sensual preferences went shopping for a new television set, one person's choice would be most influenced by what the television looked like (visual); another would be more impressed by the features as described by the salesperson (auditory); and the third shopper would only buy after being able to play with the remote control (kinesthetic).

The preference we use when we process information is likely to be our sensual preference as well. Knowing which sense you prefer makes giving yourself pleasure more intense and rewarding. It also makes relating to lovers so much simpler! For example, let's assume Jamie is a visual person. Her partner, Taylor, is kinesthetic and comes home anticipating a cuddly, sexy evening. Taylor cuddles up behind Jamie, who is working at the computer. Taylor strokes Jamie's hair and kisses her on the neck. Jamie is not seduced. In fact, Jamie finally bursts out with, "Not now. Can't you see I'm working? All you ever want is sex." Presuming Jamie and Taylor have a loving relationship and that Taylor is really not a sex maniac, what might have happened here? Taylor, being kinesthetic, approached Jamie the way Taylor would like to be approached—with touch. If Taylor had instead presented Jamie, who is visual, with a beautiful handmade card and some flowers, Jamie's reaction might have been much warmer. On the other hand, if Jamie had approached Taylor with the card and flowers instead of touch, Jamie might have gotten a similarly unenthusiastic response.

Knowing which sense you and your partner prefer simply makes giving and receiving more conscious. It's like knowing your partner's favorite color. Given the choice, wouldn't you buy pink flowers instead of yellow if you knew your partner preferred pink? And given the choice, wouldn't you rather receive the kind of erotic attention that really turns you on? Here's an exercise designed to help you pinpoint your primary sensual preference.

Try to imagine or recall each of the following items:

SIGHT

* Visualize the largest drinking glass in your kitchen cupboard.
* Recall the interior of the last car you rode in.
* See your favorite flower in bloom.
* Visualize the spots on a leopard.
* Which of your friends wears the brightest-colored clothes?
* See your favorite actor on a movie screen wearing a very revealing bathing suit.

SOUND

* Hear a dog barking in the distance.
* Hear a car alarm right outside your door.
* Recall the voice of your favorite grade-school teacher.
* Listen to a familiar melody.
* Hear rustling leaves in the trees over your head.
* Listen to water falling into a metal pail.

TOUCH

* Feel the rim of a cup of hot tea on your lips.
* Pull on a wet bathing suit.
* Stroke a long haired cat.
* Jump into a pile of leaves.
* Leap into a warm pool.
* Hold a handful of glass marbles.

SMELL

* Recall the fragrance of your mother's perfume.
* Smell leaves burning.
* Smell coffee brewing.
* Recall the aroma of your school lunch room.
* Smell a wet dog.
* Inhale the scent of a rose.

TASTE

* Suck on a lemon.
* Taste a strawberry.
* Taste burnt toast.
* Taste a mouthful of salt water.
* Taste hot salsa.
* Recall the taste of a rubber band.

So, which set of sensory memories or imaginings came most quickly and easily to you? Which set(s) took longer to imagine or seemed vague? Which sets of sensory memories triggered the most emotional or physical responses in you? The category that comes most easily and is most specific for you is your primary sensory preference.

You may have noticed that another category came in a close second. It is equally useful to make note of your secondary sensory preference. Often this secondary sense will call your attention to something, and then your primary sense will take over. For instance, I am primarily kinesthetic, and secondarily visual. If I am shopping, my eye may spot a pretty colored sweater, but then I'll have to go over and touch it. Although the color may draw me to the sweater, I will decide whether to buy it based on how it feels. Going back to our previous example with

A Science of Senses

If the science and practice of all this sensory work fascinates you, you may want to delve more deeply into Neuro-Linguistic Programming (NLP). NLP deals with the way we filter, through our five senses, our experiences of the outside world, and how we use those same senses (both intentionally and unintentionally) to achieve the results we desire. NLP was developed in the mid-1970s by John Grinder, a professor at UC Santa Cruz, and Richard Bandler, a graduate student. NLP was based on the work of Virginia Satir, a family therapist; Fritz Perls, founder of Gestalt therapy; Gregory Bateson, anthropologist; and Milton Erickson, hypnotist. It began as an exploration of the relationship between neurology, linguistics, and observable patterns ("programs") of behavior; hence the name Neuro-Linguistic Programming.

Jamie and Taylor, if Jamie were visual/kinesthetic, Taylor's approach (cuddling up behind her) would have worked, especially if the stroking and kisses were followed by a beautiful card and flowers.

How do you discover other people's preferences? You can hand them a copy of our little quiz here; or, if that's not possible or appropriate, you can simply listen to how they talk. We all give clues to our preferences in the particular words and phrases we use—for example, "I get the picture," "I hear what you're saying," or "That's feels right."

Here are some phrases people use based on their sensory preferences:

> It was so close I could taste it.
> I see what you mean.
> Show me.
> In my mind's eye . . .
> That smells pretty fishy.
> Perhaps I can shed some light on this.
> It just leaves a bad taste in my mouth.
> I hear you.
> I just feel it's gonna happen that way.
> I can see it now!
> It feels like the right thing to do.
> That's a tasty outfit you're wearing!
> Sounds right to me.
> I can smell success.

If you listen carefully to how someone phrases their thought processes, you will be able to discern their sensory preferences. This works not only with lovers, but also with coworkers and friends. It can make all your relationships easier, more rewarding, and even more productive. When Annie Sprinkle and I realized that she was visual/kinesthetic and I was kinesthetic/visual, we had a much easier time setting up our group Tantra rituals. We used to argue about which was more important: how our temple looked or how comfortable it was. When we realized why we were arguing, we simply set up two teams of helpers: one to beautify the space and one to make it clean and comfy. It worked like a charm! We had much more sumptuous temples and no arguments.

When you plan your solo Tantra with your sensory preferences in mind, you can focus on your biggest turn-ons and then expand your repertoire to include new sensations. When you know your sensual preferences, you'll find it easier to answer when a partner asks what you enjoy. And when you know the preferences of your lovers, you can give them what they enjoy without the self-torture that comes with wondering if you've guessed right.

Try New Sensations

A solo Tantra ritual is a great rehearsal space for any props or activities you might want to try but don't want to try out on a partner the first time. Solo playtime is perfect for trying blindfolds, nipple clamps, anal toys, fetish videos, exotic lube, or a rubber outfit. You may find that you have a preference for certain toys in your solo rituals that you have no interest in using when you're having sex with a partner. That's just fine. My favorite solo-only indulgence is a red and gold snake-like glass dildo.

Use your mirror, or if you prefer, your video camera. I once asked workshop participants to bring whatever accessory they wanted to use in an erotic ritual. One woman brought a video camera and everyone else at the workshop immediately wanted their erotic ritual videotaped! Video cameras may challenge vibrators as the world's most popular sex toys. Practice Tantra in front of your camera; then watch the tape to improve your technique. You will absolutely thrill your inner exhibitionist.

Take Yourself on a Tantric Date

I'd like you to invite yourself out on a real date. Open your calendar and mark out an evening just for yourself. Don't even consider the possibility of canceling it. No matter how busy we might be with work or other responsibilities, when we meet a wonderful new someone, we suddenly have lots of time to spend with them. Make this date with yourself that kind of date.

Here are some suggestions:

* Plan your date in advance, or be more spontaneous.
* Dress up and take yourself out to a lovely restaurant, and then to an exhibit of erotic photographs or a sexy show.
* Go to a sex shop and pick out a new toy and a hot video.
* Go home and make yourself a delicious dinner, and then treat yourself to a luxurious erotic bath with fragrant bath oils.

* Try the Firebreath Orgasm or the Clench and Hold.
* Whatever you choose, turn off the phone, the computer and—unless your plans include the erotic video—the television.
* Light candles.
* Fill the room with your favorite scent.
* Arrange everything you might want or need so that it's within easy reach.
* Take your time.
* Be sure to allow your plans to change if your mood changes, but don't ever stand yourself up by canceling your date!
* Keep in mind your sensory preferences. If a book of erotic stories doesn't turn you on, try a self-massage with scented oil. If the bedroom isn't turning you on, try the bathroom or the kitchen.
* Whatever you choose, remember to breathe consciously. Focusing on your breath will quiet your mind and bring your attention back to your body.
* Honor whatever feelings come up as you make love to yourself. Perhaps your orgasm may turn into a crygasm or an angergasm or a gigglegasm. Allow yourself to have whatever experience your body wants to have, and know that it is perfect for you this evening.
* If you aren't feeling sexual, honor that. You might just want to cuddle up in bed with that book you've never given yourself the time to read. The purpose of this date is for you to give yourself what you really want and need. Enjoy yourself.

Medibation

Medibation is what Annie Sprinkle calls the practice of using masturbation as a meditation. When I need a spiritual practice to empty my cluttered mind and renew my tired body, I can always count on medibation.

I approach medibation the same way I approach any meditation. I focus on my breathing and on the sensations in my body. I do not let my mind drift off into fantasies. (I sometimes hold in my mind's eye a vision of something or someone to whom I would like to dedicate some sexual energy. I'll talk more about this in chapter 22, "Sex Magic.") I try not to expect any specific insight, nor do I try to achieve anything more than being completely present in the moment.

Medibation strengthens your ability to stay present and alert, and it connects your sex with your spirit. Great medibators are usually great Tantric lovers because they have learned to see the divine in themselves and thus can see the divine in their beloved.

I encourage you to medibate daily.

Evolutionary Selfloving

Contrary to 1950s sex education films, masturbation is not something we are meant to outgrow. Masturbation is something that is meant to evolve. Our selfloving changes and grows over our lifetime. Each of us has our own intensely personal and individual sexual evolution. We pass through all sorts of phases and flavors of eroticism on our journey. Some phases may be daring and dramatic; some may be subtly profound. Something that makes you incredibly hot this year may not even catch your attention five years from now. What seems gross or scary now may be your biggest passion in a decade. Wherever you are in your erotic evolution, you can create solo sexual rituals that will support you and reward you.

This isn't the end of solo Tantra; it is, in fact, only the beginning. Much in the following chapters can be adapted wholly or in part for solo play. Many of the partner exercises can be done by yourself, with a mirror. The erotic massage strokes will turn you on whether the hand touching you is yours or your partner's. Solo rituals have all the same erotic components and potential ecstasy as rituals for two or more. Whatever your path, your most reliable, faithful, and understanding partner will always be yourself.

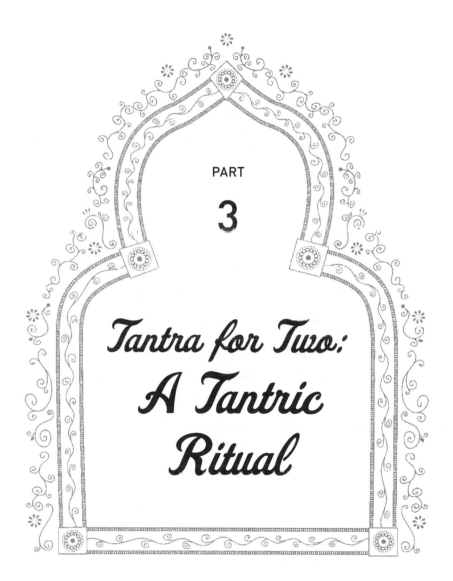

PART

3

Tantra for Two:
A Tantric
Ritual

Partner sex is usually thought of as a spontaneous expression of love and desire. Two people who are deeply in love are swept away on a wave of passion that leaves them orgasmically spent, emotionally fulfilled, and more deeply in love than ever. You just can't plan that kind of sex, right? Wrong. Preparation intensifies passion. In Tantra, planning and preparation are like foreplay. Rather than making sex seem contrived, artificial, and unsexy, preparation and planning help build erotic energy to share with a partner. In Tantra, you do not have to be in the mood for sex. Love, desire, and passion can be generated within the ritual itself.

Tantric partner sex is usually referred to as a ritual. The term *ritual* has too often been negatively used to describe events that are long, deadly dull, frightening, or just plain weird. A ritual simply separates a sacred space from the rest of life. Whether you cast a circle, gather in a special building, or simply designate a corner of a room, the space for ritual is a space set apart from everyday life for the purpose of going deeper into ourselves and raising energy in order to connect with a higher power within or without. A ritual does not have to be days or hours long, though in Tantra a long ritual can be delicious. Rituals require a clear intention and conscious preparation. What you want to accomplish with your ritual will guide you in its preparation.

In Tantra, we want to:

* Quiet the mind

* Release stress

* Energize the body

* Connect intimately with ourselves or another person or persons

* Open ourselves to the wisdom of our higher consciousness and allow ourselves to experience everything and everyone as a reflection of the Divine

A Tantric ritual can be divided into six segments, each with its own intention:

1. Set the stage: to prepare the space (see chapter 11).

2. Chill out: to relax, shake off the day, and get present (see chapter 12).

3. Warm up: to wake up your body and get your sexual energy moving (see chapter 12).

4. Come together: to connect with your partner or with your inner lover (see chapter 13).

5. Rock and roll: to enjoy some high-energy orgasmic activity (see chapter 14).

6. Afterglow: to cool down and bask in the postorgasmic ether (see chapter 15).

In this section, you will be creating each of these stages of a Tantric ritual with a partner. You'll find numerous sexual positions and exercises that fulfill the intention of each stage. You do not have to do them all at once. Try the ones that resonate most with you, and go back to the others later.

Also in this section are instructions for another type of ritual: the Erotic Awakening Massage (see chapters 16 through 18). This unique and transformative process utilizes breath, erotic touch, and breath and energy orgasm techniques in a manner that allows you to travel to unimagined heights and depths of intimacy with both yourself and your partner.

Let's begin with the first step in your ritual, setting the stage.

CHAPTER 11

Set the Stage

Doing Tantra with your partner may differ from your old style of lovemaking. At times, you may feel closer to your partner than you ever thought possible. During postures involving conscious breath, eye gazing, and movement, you may feel as though you have never met this being before. Your partner's face may seem to change. You will be more aware of the moments of merging with your partner, as well as the moments you are completely separate. This a good and natural thing. Sometimes partner sex is about the connection between the two of you; at other times you each need to go within and focus on your own experience.

At the moment of orgasm, each of you momentarily enters a realm wherein you are not only not connected to your partner, but you may not even have a sense of yourself as a separate, independent being. You may feel like pure electrical current or a thundering wave, crashing and dissolving on the shore. Your orgasm is your own experience—it is only happening to you—even though the evidence of it may be highly enjoyable for your partner to watch. You will learn to cherish your time in that solo yet connected experience as much as you'll adore the afterglow of your lovemaking which will provide all the time and space you need for reconnecting with your partner.

Preparation for this kind of deliciously intense dance goes far beyond any typical notion of foreplay. It begins with the creation of a safe, nurturing, sensual space which will support you in opening to your inner self and to your partner. In each subsequent stage of your ritual, you will be stepping incrementally deeper into the shared mystery of sexually-induced altered consciousness. You'll want your environment to enhance your experience.

We therefore begin our Tantric ritual by preparing our space. I call my Tantric ritual space "Barbara's Theatre of Sexual and Spiritual Delights" because theatre encourages a variety of environments and performances.

The Stage

Your Tantric stage is a lot more than your bed. It is at least a room and may be your entire home or, in the case of group rituals, a large rented space. How do you make your lovemaking space a sacred space? You use the same elements you'd use to create a performance space: scenery, lighting, sound, costumes, and props. Now, before you slam this book shut in frustration, breathe. This does not have to be as time-consuming as it sounds. Nor does it have to cost a lot of money. In fact, the preparation can be a lot of fun. Let me show you what I mean.

First, think like a set designer. What is the scene you are trying to create? Is it a Hindu temple? A magic cave? A vampire's lair? Another planet? Be creative! You do not have to go out and have a set built, but keeping an image in mind will make it easier and more fun to choose the elements you'll use to create your space.

Second, think about which design elements matter the most to you. Comfort? Visual beauty? Beautiful sounds? Great food? Yummy smells? You may not have time to create all of these as fully as you like, so pick what matters most to you and your partner(s). When I set up for a group ritual, my first priorities are comfort and music, so I enlist the help of other temple-builders who feel passionately about decorations and food. That way everyone gets what they want most.

Scenery

Choose a room to be your primary ritual space. Do not automatically choose the bedroom. You won't be using the bed much (if at all) during Tantra, so if your living situation permits, be more creative. You can do ecstatic Tantra in just about every room of the house. Some of my favorite rituals have made use of multiple rooms, starting with a sensuous bath in the bathroom, followed by an erotic massage in the living room, culminating with a play piercing in the parlor. What if you have only one room? No problem. I practiced Tantra for years in a tiny studio apartment. Almost all of the exercises, positions, and practices can be adapted for small spaces.

The first step to creating an ideal lovemaking space is simple but critical: clean up! Tidy your space. Get rid of clutter and dirt. A cluttered space is psychically disturbing. If you can't clear out all the clutter, at least cover it with a pretty cloth. Cover the computer, too! In Tantra, a computer screen is not a sex toy.

Place a futon, yoga mat, or some pillows or cushions on the floor. The floor is a much better Tantric space than a bed. A nice, soft mattress may feel wonderful after your ritual, but it's not conducive to staying present and awake. Besides, the floor is safer. No matter how wild you get, you can't fall off the floor. But staying present and awake doesn't mean being uncomfortable. Make sure the room temperature is right, the cushions are comfy, and you can easily change position anytime you start to feel stiff or cramped.

Decorate. Make the space pretty. Use brightly colored cloths, flowers, pretty cushions—anything that looks and feels sensuous. I've seen spaces decorated with pictures, jewelry, photos, crystals, plants, flowers, straw, ferns, fur, garlands, holiday twinkle lights, feathers, toys, leather, tinsel, and mirrors.

Lighting

Turn off the electric lights. Get back to basics: candles, candles, and more candles. Candles flicker like stars, and their light makes everyone look beautiful and feel special. I prefer the large votive candles—the ones in glass containers. They are much safer than naked candles. In the throes of ecstasy, you won't be thinking about whether your candles are behaving properly. One especially blissed out Tantrika friend of mine burned down her temple one evening when an unprotected candle made contact with a flowing decorative cloth. In Tantra, we do try to include as much of the four elements of nature—air, fire, water, and earth—as we can; but trust me, there is such a thing as too much fire energy.

Sound

Music is one of the most important parts of my Tantric rituals. Tantra does not limit you to soft, instrumental, New Age, or classical choices. I often use intense, rhythmic African drumming and Aboriginal didgeridoo, as well as schmaltzy, beautiful, heart-opening music. The keys to choosing your music are rhythm and flow. Does the music make you want to move? Good!

How does it make you move? Is the music energy-building, or is it relaxing? Does the music open your heart and relax your shoulders? Does it make you want to move your hips? Hard, soft, fast, and slow sounds all have a place in your ritual, as well as sounds that transport you to another realm. Try space music or recordings of thunderstorms or raging oceans. Gather a juicy selection and have it close at hand so that you can change your music as you change your mood.

Do not choose heavy metal or rap music with violent lyrics (a.k.a. gansta rap) in your rituals—not even for intense energy building. Tantra does not have many hard-and-fast rules, so I expect you to really pay attention to the few I insist on. Tantra is designed to open up all your energy centers and allow love and consciousness to flow through you. The energy—not to mention the often violent lyrics—of heavy metal and gansta rap music is psychically and physically depleting, and you just do not want that much violence and negativity around you when you are in such an open state. If you want a strong, fast beat, there are plenty of healthier choices available, such as Babatunde Olatunji's *Drums of Passion* series. In addition, be mindful of music with lyrics. Make sure the lyrics are loving and positive and affirming, not doom-and-gloom. I generally use music without lyrics, or music with chanting or lyrics in a language I do not understand.

Am I saying that you should never listen to heavy metal or gangsta rap? No. I like rap and hip-hop. I simply stay away from violent and misogynistic lyrics. I enjoy my occasional shot of Nirvana or Marilyn Manson. I just never play it in Tantric ritual spaces.

Costumes

Think like a theatrical costume designer. In the theatre, a costume not only has to look beautiful, it also has to be practical. Can you breathe deeply in it? Can you move and dance in it? Can you sit comfortably? Does it come off easily? Not surprisingly, Tantra favors sarongs and other loose, flowing costumes rather than tightly laced corsets. However, the style of your costume can be as kinky as you like, so long as it does not inhibit your ability to build sexual energy with breath and movement. When it comes to looking and feeling sexy, try to think outside the box. If you always wear lingerie, try a sarong. If you always dress like a goddess, try a touch of slut. Happily, a number of designers of latex and leather clothing are now embracing comfort and mobility, so you can be a kinky Tantrika if you like. Just make sure you can breathe and move freely!

Props

Which props to use (and whether to use them at all) is a matter of personal taste. In my rituals, I always include both hard and soft sex toys, as well as a generous selection of dildos and vibrators. As we will see, it does not matter so much which toys you use, but rather how consciously you use them.

Traditionally, Tantric toys and tantalizers have tended to be softer—for example, feathers, fur, satin, chocolate, fruit, whipped cream, essential oils, and massage oils. But there is plenty of room for toys that produce more intense sensations, such as floggers and needles. Toys are not the focus of Tantra, they are tools—just like breath, movement, imagination, sound, and Kegels. Props may be sorted according to the type of sensation they produce. Your choice of props answers the question "What do I want to feel right now?" or "Which sensation will open me up so I can feel more?"

On the opposite page is a table of props, divided into groups based on the type of sensations they provide, from subtle to severe, and graded from mild to wild.

Do you see what I mean about a range of sensations? Don't worry if you have never heard of some of these items or would never consider using them erotically. The point of identifying all these possibilities is not to get you to go out and buy a lot of props; nor am I asking you to experiment with props that can be dangerous if you don't know exactly how to play with them. But if any of the "wilder" items listed above sound like fun to you, read chapter 19 now, and by all means check out these toys in a good BDSM reference book (see the Resources section in this book) or on the Internet. Then seek out proper instruction from an experienced player before you use them. The "milder" props, like the Tingler and the ball massager, can be found in many metaphysical catalogs.

Start thinking about what kinds of sensations you are most fond of and what degrees of intensity you might enjoy. And guess what—you have dozens of unexplored sensation-creating devices in every room of your house at this very moment.

To give yourself an idea of what's available, try this: Go into your kitchen and select six cooking utensils at random. Invent a way to use each one as a sex toy. (Please don't write me with any suggestions for the food processor or toaster oven. I don't want to know.) What sensation—or range of sensations—can you produce with each item?

The fun doesn't stop with utensils. Try this exercise with food: Have you ever sculpted yourself a veggie dildo? Carrots work very well. So do zucchinis and other squash. Pick a vegetable that's close to the size and shape you prefer, and perfect it a bit with a knife. (Caution: some vegetables can get a bit unstable if carved too drastically.) Be creative!

Props: Mild to Wild

	MILD	▶ ▶ ▶ ▶ ▶	▶ ▶ ▶ ▶ ▶	▶ ▶ ▶ ▶ ▶	WILD
SOFT	Feathers	Fur	Whipped cream	Jell-O	Mud
COOL	Breath	Fruit juice	Ice cream	Tile floor	Ice
HOT	Breath	Hot tub	Heat rub	Candle wax	Branding iron
SHARP	Long fingernails	Quills (*sharp end of a feather*)	Talons[4]	Needles (*for play piercings, permanent piercings, or tattooing*)	Scalpels
PINCHY	Fingers	Pickle tongs	Ice tongs	Nipple clamps	Clothespins[6]
THUDDY	Pillows	Ball massagers[3]	Boxing gloves	Socks filled with rice	Floggers[7]
TINGLY	The Tingler[1]	Motel bed with "Magic Fingers"	Vibrators	Violet wands[5]	TENS units[8]
STINGING	Slapping with palm of hand	Snapping rubber bands	Wooden spoons	Paddles	Single-tail whips
DARK OR SILENT	Blindfolds	Earplugs	Masks	Gags	Hoods
TIGHT (*a.k.a. restraint or light bondage*)	Licorice whips[2]	Velcro wrist cuffs	Police handcuffs	Corseting	Duct tape over plastic wrap over petroleum jelly
SLIPPERY	Satin	Massage with cornstarch	Massage with oil	Full-body massage with tongue	Wrestling in salad oil

1. The Tingler is a copper-fingered head massager designed to stimulate the nerves and acupressure points of the scalp.
2. Licorice whips are two- to three-foot-long strings of candy that make edible bondage ropes.
3. A ball massager is a rubber ball mounted on a flexible metal or plastic handle.
4. Talons are sharp, pointed metal claws that fit over the tips of your fingers. They can be used for a wide range of sensations, from tickling and stroking to deep scratching and clawing.
5. A violet wand is an electrical unit that produces an arc of static electricity. It produces a purely surface sensation.
6. Clothespins aren't as innocent as they look. The longer you leave them on the skin, the more they hurt when they come off.
7. A flogger is a whip with multiple wide, flat tails.
8. A TENS (transcutaneous electrical nerve stimulator) unit is a device that sends an actual surge of electricity deeper into the muscles.

Special Effects

One Tantric tradition I have always loved is the inclusion of the four elements of nature—air, fire, water, and earth in each ritual. Those of us in urban environments are nature-starved. The act of collecting and acknowledging the four elements is soothing to the soul. Be sure to include at least one item representing each element. Some items contain more than one element, making your job even easier.

Air. Make sure your space is properly ventilated. Open a window. Even if it is cold outside, you can still open the window a crack. You'll be doing a lot of breathing. When you get lightheaded, it should be because your consciousness has been altered by erotic energy—not by lack of oxygen! Seriously, lack of fresh air will cause you to space out and lose focus on yourself and your partner(s).

Fire. You don't have to have a fireplace. Candles will do very nicely. Just use sensible safety precautions. Burning incense is also nice, and it brings in an earth element as well.

Water. You'll want water for drinking and bathing. You might also like earth water (fruit juice), air water (sparkling mineral water), earth-fire water (wine), or my favorite, combining all the elements in one: earth-air-fire water (champagne). Just be careful of the fire waters. A few sips build fire (sexual) energy, but a few glasses drain it away completely.

Earth. The most popular earth element for a Tantric ritual is food. There are unlimited ways to be sexy with food. When you plan the food for your ritual, choose food that is both sexy and nourishing for you. Many people like fruit. It's sweet and tasty, and satisfies your thirst. However, some people, myself included, just can't handle that much sugar. I need to have a bit of cheese or some other kind of protein along with it. What food does your body need in high-energy situations? (Whenever I ask this question in workshops, the nearly unanimous answer is invariably, *"Chocolate!"*)

Other earth elements that help make a great ritual are flowers; natural or sculpted objects of wood or stone; crystals; and scents such as amber, musk, sandalwood, ylang-ylang, and patchouli. You can use essential oils and an aromatherapy burner, or light sticks or cones of incense.

Safer Sex

It was my desire for an ecstatic sexual practice that included safer sex that originally led me to Tantra. Preparation and consciousness are necessary for both safer sex and Tantric sex. Condoms and gloves will in no way diminish your sexual enjoyment because Tantra focuses on charging the entire body—not just the genitals—with sexual energy, making your entire body a pulsing, tingling, vibrating sex organ.

Make a personal decision about which safer sex practices you are going to practice. Safer sex means sexual activity with no exchange of bodily fluids. Bodily fluids include ejaculate (male or female), blood (including menstrual blood), vaginal secretions, urine, feces, and the discharges from sores caused by sexually transmitted infections. "No exchange" means that none of the bodily fluids of one partner ever gets into the vagina, penis, anus, mouth, eyes, nose, or open skin wounds of another.

Safer-sex protocol is necessary when either you or your partner have any sexually transmitted disease (STD), including—and this is the important part—when you aren't sure. Unless you are in a strictly monogamous relationship with someone whose HIV/STD status you are certain of, you need to know about and practice safer sex.

Not only is HIV as prevalent as it ever was, but there are also a host of other sexually transmitted diseases out there. Some can be with you for a lifetime. That's why safer sex is now commonly defined as anything one does to lower the risks of getting or giving any sexually transmitted disease. Think of safer sex as a spectrum: some behaviors are riskier than others. Think about which sexual activities you find the most pleasurable. Then take into account the risks involved and whether any of those will worry you later. Last, think about how you can lower the risks while increasing your pleasure. Do all this before you engage in any intimate behavior.

You may be thinking that safer sex is something you just don't have to worry about. Perhaps you have been with the same partner for years. Or perhaps your only sex partner is yourself right now. Nevertheless, please read the following section. As you go further into Tantra, you may find that you want to explore something new. That new

How Safe Is Safe?

When the AIDS epidemic exploded in the early/mid 1980s, anyone who was sexually active was forced to choose between practicing safer sex and the very real possibility of contracting a fatal illness. AIDS was considered 100 percent fatal at that time, and the only way to be sexual and be sure that you weren't going to get AIDS was to follow the strictest safer sex guidelines to the letter. Even tears and saliva were considered possible transmitters of the virus. Over time, we have learned that there is not enough HIV present in tears and saliva to transmit the virus, and we have adjusted safer sex guidelines accordingly. But now that people are not dying by the hundreds every day—in this country—many people have gotten more casual about safer sex practices. This is a big mistake and, in some cases, borders on criminal negligence.

something or someone may present the need to make a new decision about safer sex. The time to make safer-sex decisions is before you take your clothes off.

Everyone should have a basic safe-sex supply kit within easy reach. You don't need a lot of stuff to play safely. The following few essential basics will do.

CONDOMS

Use latex condoms for all intercourse—vaginal or anal. They help protect against gonorrhea, syphilis, chlamydia, herpes, hepatitis B, and AIDS. To be effective, condoms should be put on during foreplay, before there is any preejaculatory fluid. After intercourse, withdraw the penis while it is still hard, and remove the condom carefully. It's important to grasp the base of the condom during withdrawal so that the condom doesn't slip off.

Use condoms on your sex toys, if you share them. They work on dildos, anal plugs, and vibrators. Use a new condom for each partner who uses the toy. Never reuse a condom.

For oral sex, use a nonlubricated or flavored condom. A word of warning: condoms lubricated with Nonoxynol-9 taste terrible! You can also cut a condom lengthwise, open it up, and place it over the anus or vulva for oral-anal sex (rimming) or oral-vaginal sex (cunnilingus).

LUBE

Use plenty of water-based lube (such as Astroglide, ID, ForPlay, Wet, or Probe) on the outside of the condom for comfort and mutual pleasure, and to keep the condom from tearing during sex. Some men find that more sensation is transmitted to them if they put a small amount of water- or silicone-based lube inside the tip of their condom before putting it on. Use only water- or silicone-based lubricants on condoms. Oil-based lubricants, such as Vaseline, Crisco, and hand lotions, weaken latex and make condoms break.

GLOVES

Do you need to wear gloves before you touch someone's pussy, ass, or cock? Here's how you tell: cut a lemon in half and rub it all over your hands and fingers. (Vinegar works as well as lemons.) If you feel any stinging, you have breaks in your skin that could let germs enter or exit your bloodstream. Glove up! You can buy either latex or vinyl gloves at a drugstore or medical supply store. If you want to do anal play (including fisting) with an oil-based lube (which some people prefer), be sure to get vinyl gloves. Vinyl is not compromised by oil the way latex is.

I know the idea of wearing gloves during sex can seem weird. But I swear they can be sexy. I know women who get wet just hearing the snap of a latex glove. Try both vinyl and latex. Many people have a strong preference for the feel of one over the other.

PLASTIC WRAP

Plain old plastic food wrap is the best barrier for rimming and cunnilingus. Do not use the microwaveable kind, as it has little holes in it that defeat the purpose of a barrier. You can roll out a piece of plastic wrap large enough to cover both the vulva and anus. It's much easier to hang on to than a cut-open condom, and it's a lot thinner than a dental dam. Spread some lube on your partner's side of the plastic wrap for increased sensation. Just make sure that the plastic wrap doesn't touch the anus and then the vulva. Germs passed from anus to vagina can cause a nasty infection.

Some people do prefer dental dams for oral sex, but I find them too thick and too hard to hold on to. It's easy to drop a dam when it gets slippery, and then you may not be able to tell which side has been against the body.

SPECIAL SITUATIONS

The following situations present special issues relating to safer sex.

Oral sex. Some people feel that safer-sex barriers are not as necessary for oral sex as they are for vaginal and anal sex. I disagree. Yes, it's clear that the risk of transmitting HIV is much lower for unprotected oral sex than for unprotected anal or vaginal intercourse. But this is not true for transmission of herpes, gonorrhea, syphilis, and chlamydia. And the risk of transmitting all these STDs is greater if you have any open sores in your mouth. I'm prone to chewing the inside of my lip when I'm worried, and my periodontist is none too thrilled about my gums, so I'm not going to go down on someone without a barrier.

The female condom. The female condom is a plastic sheath that women can insert into their vaginas for use in protection against HIV and STDs. The female condom can be inserted up to eight hours before sex, has rings at both ends to hold it in place, and can be lubricated with oil-based lubricants, which stay wet longer than the water-based variety. This kind of condom takes practice to use, and it's more expensive than a latex condom. Some men have also used the female condom for anal sex, though I've not heard of any tests done to prove them safe for this use.

Water sports. It's safe to urinate on skin without open cuts or sores. Use the lemon/vinegar test. Urine that enters the mouth, vagina, or rectum is not safe. It could spread HIV or hepatitis B.

Blood sports. Serious aficionados of piercings, cuttings, or any kind of blood sports know that the lighting has to be bright, the instruments sterile, and the protocol impeccable to keep everyone safe. Any of these more arcane pleasure techniques, done incorrectly, could result in permanent injury or transmission of serious disease. You'll need to learn both the techniques and the hygienic protocol from an experienced person. Merely seeing it done once or twice at a play party is not enough! Ask an experienced player to teach you how to do things safely and with maximum pleasure.

Troubleshooting. What happens when something goes wrong—if the condom breaks, or you realize you forgot to put on your gloves after your hand is inside your lover? Don't freak, just fix it. Your first step in getting back on the safer-sex track is washing up. Wash your hands, your toys, your genitals, and whatever you can with antibacterial soap. If that's not appropriate (for instance, if you got some cum in your eyes), just wash with lots of water.

What if a condom fails during vaginal or anal intercourse? If it is still inside the vagina or anus, immediately remove the condom. The receptive partner shouldn't douche; that might increase the likelihood of infection. If any Nonoxynol-9 contraceptive foam is handy, it might help to insert it and leave it in for about fifteen minutes. Nonoxynol-9 can kill HIV, but several clinical studies show that it does not prevent HIV infection, and may actually increase the risk of infection in women, presumably by inflaming and damaging vaginal tissues. Nonoxynol-9 has been shown to provide some protection against gonorrhea and chlamydia. Men can give themselves a little extra protection after potential exposure to an STD by immediately visiting the restroom, urinating, and then washing their genitals with an antibacterial soap.

Remember: While practicing safer sex dramatically reduces the risk of contracting or passing on the most serious sexually transmitted ailments, it does not completely eliminate the risk for every possible condition.

Tantric sex can be completely safe sex. You can combine energy sex with masturbation and have a mind-, body-, and spirit-altering experience without the risk of exchanging a single bodily fluid. If you are practicing safer sex, plan it in advance. Make it part of your preparation. Then practice it as slowly and consciously as you would any other element of your ritual.

This chapter is intended to make you aware of all the possible elements in your environmet that can enhance (or detract from) your erotic pleasure. Use this chapter as a reference guide, not as a ritual setup bible. You do not have to do everything I have suggested in each section. You do, however, want to set up an attractive, safe, clean space that invites your senses to open up and take in more colors, smells, feelings, sounds, and tastes. Not only will the resulting environment enhance your pleasure, but the act of setting up your ritual stage will prepare your mind for the pleasure to come.

CHAPTER 12

Chill Out and Warm Up

Now that you have prepared your space, it is time to prepare *you* for your Tantric ritual. This preparation need not take the better part of a day. You may not have hours to devote to cleaning and decorating your space prior to a long, luxurious process of bathing, meditating, and dressing ceremoniously. What's important is that you make a tangible transition between your everyday life and your erotic life. You need to complete this transition before trying to connect with your partner. If time constraints force a choice between preparing your space and preparing yourself, put the emphasis on yourself. Quickly tidy up the ritual space. Light some candles and a stick of incense. Gather safer-sex supplies and any sensual delights you plan to use. Then spend your time on you.

Chill Out

First, empty yourself of physical, mental, and psychic gunk—the kind we all accumulate as we go through our daily lives. Relax your tensed body, calm your racing mind, and reconnect with your spirit. In other words, love yourself before making love. Here are some tips for how to do this:

Cleanse yourself. Take a bath or a shower. Make sure the water is not too hot, and don't stay too long—a long, hot bath will drain too much fire energy and leave you too relaxed. Burn some sage in a metal bowl and bathe yourself in the smoke to cleanse your psychic body and auric field.

Clear out emotional gunk. Scream underwater or into a pillow. Throw a few karate chops, chopping away anything you're angry about or preoccupied with. Do the Exhilaration Meditation or Cathartic Meditation (see chapter 4), or an abbreviated version of one of them. You could even do just one section of either. Shaking for just five or ten minutes will help clear out the cobwebs and help you to be more present.

Change your outfit. Follow the advice of my enlightened drag queen sisters: "Change your clothes, change your consciousness." Change into something—whether it's a silk sarong or a rubber cat suit—that tells your body it's time to feel sexy.

Warm Up

After you have prepared yourself to meet your partner (who has similarly prepared), it's time to warm up together to ready each other for sex. Here are some exercises and techniques to help you wake up your body and ignite your erotic energy. One of the easiest and nicest ways to start is with a great hug.

Grounding Hug

First you will give the hug, then you will receive it.

1. Stand with your feet hip-distance apart and your knees slightly bent. Breathe using the Bottom Breath (see chapter 4), bringing your awareness to your root chakra. Imagine that your legs are huge, strong tree roots anchoring you deep into the earth.
2. Now embrace your partner. Place one hand on their lower back, and the other on their upper/middle back. Breathe your belly into their belly. As you hug, imagine that you are grounding your partner in the earth, rooting them the way you are rooted.
3. Continue to breathe together, feeling your partner letting go and relaxing. You will actually feel your partner's center of gravity move down into their pelvis and legs.
4. Switch positions; now it's your turn to receive. Receive the grounding hug with as much consciousness as you gave it.

✳
Partner Shake

If you and your partner don't feel like doing the shaking portion of the Exhilaration Meditation by yourselves, you can always shake each other. It works out the kinks and it has just the right silliness quotient.

1. Vibrate your partner, starting at the top of their head and working your way down their body. The vibrations don't have to be hard, but they should be fairly rapid. Go gently on the head; be more vigorous on the arms, hands, buttocks, and legs.
2. Switch places; it's your turn to receive.

✳
Elephant Massage

1. Your partner (the elephant) stands with feet hip-distance apart, bending forward from the waist, arms hanging down like an elephant's trunk. Elephant masseur/masseuse, you can stand behind your elephant or in front—whichever is more comfortable for you.
2. Now give your partner an elephant massage. How do you massage an elephant? Any way the elephant wants, of course! But I'd suggest you concentrate on those tense elephant shoulders and tight elephant spine. Elephant, you can sway your trunk back and forth if you like and make appreciative elephant sounds when your masseur gets it just right.
3. As you complete your massage, step directly behind and very close to your elephant. Let them roll up, vertebra by vertebra, leaning against you, until their head is leaning back on your shoulder. After a few moments, help them to stand on their own.
4. Now, elephant masseur, it's your turn to be the elephant.

✳
Activate the Microcosmic Orbit

1. Your partner stands with feet hip-distance apart. Placing their awareness at their perineum, they breathe in, drawing energy around and up to their tailbone, up their spine and neck, over the top of their head, and finally down their forehead to the roof of

their mouth. As they do this, trace this pathway (the back channel) with your hand, tapping all along the spine, up to the top of their head.

2. Your partner then places the tip of their tongue on the roof of their mouth and exhales, letting the energy trickle down the front of their body, down to their genitals and back to their perineum. As they exhale, brush down this pathway (the front channel) with your fingers.

3. Repeat until your partner feels the Microcosmic Orbit as an actual circuit of energy.

4. Now switch places with your partner.

Your intention in this section of your ritual is to release any stress and tension you felt prior to the start of the ritual and replace it with a relaxed, alive awareness. The exercises above are suggestions. Create your own techniques. Laugh for ten minutes. Wrestle with your partner. Have a pillow fight. Any activity that leaves you relaxed but tingly and ready for more is perfect.

CHAPTER 13

Come Together

In these next three chapters, you will learn several traditional Tantric lovemaking positions and—just as important—variations that will help personalize and add variety to your ritual. I hope they will also give you some ideas for creating your own variations. As you try each posture, I suggest you start off with the traditional form and then allow it to morph into one or more of the variations. This way, you'll get a sense of the original intent and also find the form that works best for you and your partner.

Tantric lovemaking positions allow you to build, share, and circulate sexual energy with a partner. In the process of a Tantric ritual, you will circulate two distinct expressions of life/sex energy: the genital/sexual/lower chakra energy and the heart/spiritual/upper chakra energy. During lovemaking, you'll want to keep both fires lit and burning brightly. If all the heat is in your genitals, you will miss the presence of the Divine within you both. If all the heat is in your heart and upper chakras, you will miss the passion and desire for each other. Many of the postures can be done with or without genital contact or penetration. You can add actual fucking where and when you like.

The Pose of Recognition with Hand Balancing

When we first come together with a partner, we want to open up and invite our partner into our emotional and physical space in the same way we are welcomed into theirs. In order to do this, we need to drop our emotional and physical defenses. This pose helps us to feel less separate by harmonizing our energy with our partner's.

The Pose of Recognition with hand balancing is most easily done on the floor. Use pillows to make yourselves comfortable. Sit directly across from one another, close but not quite touching, with your legs crossed. Look into your partner's nondominant eye. (If you are right-handed, your left eye is your nondominant eye; if you're left-handed, it's your right eye.) Put your right hand, palm down, onto your partner's upturned left hand. Put your left hand, palm up, under your partner's downturned right hand.

It is said that the eyes are the gateway to the soul. Tantrikas believe that the non-dominant eye is the receptive eye, and therefore the actual gateway to the soul. It is not necessary to keep your gaze glued to your partner's eye—but eye gazing is a wonderfully intimate practice, and it does give you a very specific place to put your gaze. This helps to keep your attention focused.

Traditionally, the hand balancing exercise helps to unite your yang/masculine energy (situated on the right side of your body) with your yin/feminine energy (located on the left side of your body) by joining with the opposite polarities of your partner. The upturned hand receives love; the downturned hand projects love.

Some people like to invoke the Tantric love god, Shiva, and the goddess, Shakti, by calling or singing their names. You can simply gaze into your partner's eye and recognize the god/goddess/divinity in them. You'll see your own divinity reflected back to you.

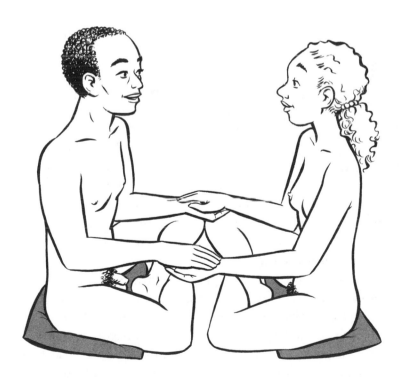

The Pose of Recognition

VARIATIONS ON THE POSE OF RECOGNITION

Feel free to modify the Pose of Recognition so that it meets your physical, emotional, and physical needs. Here are some suggestions.

Sitting positions. Instead of sitting directly in front of each other, sit slightly to the side of each other and gently hold hands. Sitting directly in front of each other can feel confrontational to people who are used to facing off across a desk with a boss or a competitor. The last thing we need at the beginning of lovemaking is to feel confrontational!

> **A Note to the Time-Challenged**
>
> Yes, it will certainly take longer than twenty minutes to practice all these positions. But it will only take twenty minutes to practice one or two of them. Eventually, you may want to make the time to string them all together in a ritual. But, please, do start enjoying at least some of them right now. Simply add one or two to whatever kind of erotic play you're already enjoying. If you wait until you have the time to do all of these, you may never try any of them.

Leg positions. You can use a wide variety of leg positions for all the sitting postures. Don't feel that you have to sit in the classic cross-legged lotus position unless it's comfortable for you. You can sit on a pillow or two so that your knees are lower than your hips, with your legs outstretched over your partner's outstretched legs. You can even sit on chairs. The most important thing is that you both be comfortable. If at any time you feel uncomfortable, move! Change positions. Staying conscious during sex means first and foremost knowing and responding to what your body is feeling. You cannot be totally present when you're sore or cramping!

Hand balancing. Hand balancing is traditionally used to balance male and female energies. I look at this somewhat differently. For me, hand balancing helps balance all my identities, not just male and female—or even yin and yang. When I feel out of balance, it's not my male and female sides that need balancing—it's all the other identities I try to juggle on a daily basis!

Living in the Western world at the beginning of this millennium means not living one life, but ninety-nine lives. We become more people in one day than our ancestors were in a lifetime. Here are just some of the identities that I've been juggling while writing this book: author, Broadway theatre manager, sex educator, workshop facilitator, friend, daughter of two parents in their late eighties, gardener, herbalist, meditator, artist, and lover. I also went from caregiver to estate executrix when an old and dear friend of mine became seriously ill and died.

So, when I sit down opposite my lover and connect with her in the hand balancing position, I'm not focused on balancing male and female. I want to balance all my identities and, specifically, bring the lover identity into proper balance. It is the myself-as-lover who gets pushed aside and buried by busyness and the demands made on me by all my other identities.

This may in fact be the primary reason why so many people who are truly in love with each other are not making love to each other. Their inner lover has been shoved aside by all the other identities a person needs to be in a day. Use hand balancing to bring your inner lover in balance with all your other identities.

Imagine that in your left hand, you hold yourself as Lover. In your right hand, you hold all your other identities. Put your right hand, palm down, onto your partner's upturned left hand (which holds their self as Lover). Put your left hand, palm up, under your partner's downturned right hand. Let your identities flow.

Drawing in the sacred. Tantric practice includes seeing the god/dess in your partner or calling your partner a god/dess. This works for many people, but not for all of us. I consider myself a very spiritual person, but I'm uncomfortable seeing my partner as either a conduit for, or the literal incarnation of, an anthropomorphized deity.

A healthy compromise might be the twelve-step model of a higher power. You can decide for yourself who or what your higher power is. One friend of mine, an atheist and recovering alcoholic, decided her higher power would be the singer Robert Goulet. Whenever she wanted a drink she called upon Robert Goulet to keep her from drinking. It worked for her; she's still sober. Your higher power could be a God, a Goddess, the Universe, All That Is, Source, the Divine, an energy force, an inner knowing, or Dolly Parton.

I believe that all human desire for connection is really a desire for connection with some higher power—a desire for a connection to something greater than our everyday selves. Relationships, especially sexual relationships, provide an ideal arena in which to practice and enjoy connection. The act of raising sexual/life-force energy in any situation puts us in closer connection with our higher power. Add a partner and the effect is multiplied. Therefore, it makes sense that when we raise sexual energy while connecting with a partner, we feel or see the presence of a higher power reflected in that partner—hence the Tantric tradition of seeing God/dess in your partner.

Communication. The Pose of Recognition is a good position for sharing anything that needs or wants to be spoken so that the two of you can move deeper into erotic intimacy. If you are with a new partner, each of you can ask and answer "How do you like to be touched?" If you have been partners for a while, each of you can ask and answer "What are some things you love about me?" If you'll be moving from this position into an activity that requires consent and negotiation, each of you can tell the other what you would like to do, might like to do, and definitely would not like to do.

Should you feel the need to clear out some feelings that you think may be preventing you from opening up to your partner, or if you are feeling emotionally stuck, you can each complete a little exercise to help you get in touch with what you are feeling.

> *I am angry about . . .*
> *I am sad about . . .*
> *I am scared about . . .*
> *I am glad about . . .*

This is not a discussion or a bitch session; it's an emotional clearing exercise. Complete all four statements without interruption or comment by your partner. Then allow your partner to do the same. Repeat until you can move ahead in peace. You will probably discover that whatever is making your partner mad, sad, glad, or scared has nothing to do with you. If anything does come up that might merit further discussion, agree to set it aside to discuss later if it's still on your mind.

Other suggestions. As you do eye gazing and hand balancing, you may feel a desire to reach out toward your partner and pull them toward you. Please resist that temptation. You don't have to do anything except breathe. Just be with them and with yourself. See what happens. Feel what comes up. Just be.

The Pose of Giving and Receiving

I can always count on the Pose of Giving and Receiving to drop me into my body and restore my ability to receive pleasure. When you give the strokes at the Resilient Edge of Resistance, you'll find giving as pleasurable as receiving.

Sit across from one another. One partner sits with their hands resting on their thighs, palms up. This person is the receiver. The receiver does not give out energy; he or she accepts it.

First stroke. The giver begins at the top of the receiver's head and, slowly and gently, like a feather, strokes down the receiver's head, neck, shoulders, arms, and wrists, and finally off the hands. Do this once.

Second stroke. The giver again begins at the top of his or her partner's head, but now strokes down to the third eye (center of the forehead), lightly strokes the receiver's eyes, moves back to the ears, comes forward and touches the nose with his or her thumbs, brings the thumbs down to the lips, and then strokes down the chin to the throat center. The giver continues stroking down to the receiver's heart center; brushes the nipples, outer torso, and inner thighs; moves back to the wrists; and slowly moves off the hands and fingertips.

Third stroke. The second stroke is repeated.

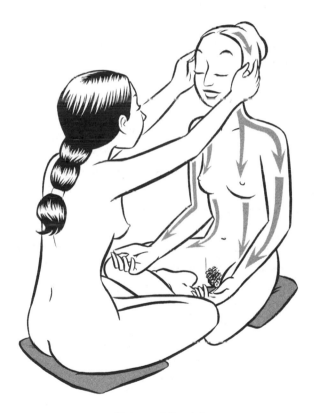

Giving and Receiving

The giver then turns his or her attention inward and becomes the receiver, placing palms upward on thighs as his or her partner becomes the giver, stroking down the receiver's body three times. Remember to go *slowly*—you cannot do this stroke too slowly. And breathe, both of you.

One purpose of this exercise is to learn to go totally into receiving when you are receiving, and totally into giving when you are giving. While doing this exercise, notice which role is more difficult for you—giving or receiving. Allow yourself the balance of being able to relate in both ways.

VARIATIONS ON GIVING AND RECEIVING

Once you've gotten used to doing this pose in the traditional manner, try experimenting with some variations.

Add a more intense touch. Do the first stroke in the traditional manner. Use your fingertips and be as soft and delicate as you can. For the second and third strokes, use your fingernails, or ice, or even the tines of a fork. For these more intense strokes, you may have to change the path you follow. For instance, ice would be harmless if stroked over the face, neck, and inner arms, but if you wanted to use a fork (or something even sharper, such as a talon), you might start at the tops of the shoulders and stroke down the outsides of the arms, avoiding prominent veins, nerve centers, and tendons.

Do the strokes on the back. This is safer and more appropriate for sharp items and many other intense sensations. Stroke down your partner's arms or back, to their buttocks. Or, start with your fingers on their head and neck, and then switch to the sharp item when you reach their upper arms.

Have the receiver lie down. This way you can stroke your partner from the top of their head to the tip of their toe. You can use light, delicate strokes on their front; then have them turn over, and use more intense strokes on their back.

Add bondage. Here's a little nugget of Taoist wisdom: sensory deprivation amplifies chi by conserving it. When you blindfold someone, chi cannot leak out their eyes. When you use earplugs, chi can't leak out their ears. Having more chi means having more energy. This is how sensory deprivation intensifies sensation, making your strokes even more delectable.

Add food. Feed your partner a morsel of chocolate or fruit between strokes. Run the morsel over their lips and tongue, but don't let them bite it yet. Allow them to experience the aroma, the texture, and the temperature of the food, and only then let them have a small bite. Go slowly; don't let them gobble it.

The Garden of Sensual Delights

This giving-and-receiving ritual focuses on opening the senses. It can be done as part of a longer Tantric ritual or on its own. It can be an inventive and intimate game to play with a new lover or with someone you're not ready to have genital sex with. It's also a great exercise for rekindling desire between lovers who've grown bored by repetitive, unconscious sex.

First, you will give to your partner, and then you'll repeat the exercise receiving from your partner. The receiver is blindfolded. Placing the receiver in bondage can also be delightful. (This can be achieved by means of real physical restraints or simply a verbal command not to move a muscle.) Just make sure that the only sense completely blocked out for the entire exercise is sight. If you want to play with gags or earplugs, remove them for the taste or auditory portions of the exercise.

PREPARATION

Separately, you and your partner go through your respective homes and gather items that you can use to delight and stimulate each other's senses. Do this separately so that neither of you knows what delights lie in store. Some suggestions for each of the senses follow:

* *Taste*: chocolate, fruit, mustard, whipped cream, salsa, a sparkling beverage, a few granules of salt, diluted lemon juice, sweet or sour pickles
* *Smell*: essential oils, a flower, mothballs, kitchen spices, motor oil, rich garden soil, your skin, a blown-out match, tuna fish
* *Touch*: a feather; a silk or satin scarf; a cold, smooth stone; sandpaper; leather; your fingernails; chain links; a warm (but not scalding) cup of tea
* *Sound*: bells, drums, wind chimes, the rattle of chains, whistles, pebbles dropped one by one into a glass of water, your whisper, a cat purring

This is meant to be a fun and pleasurable adventure. Avoid sensory cues that you know your partner dislikes, but do try to be creative in your choices. A warm (or cool) washcloth on the back of the neck is a wonderful sensation when you are blindfolded. So is the sound of singing through a vacuum cleaner hose. Don't forget that some of your selections will have multiple sensual properties (for example, leather has a distinctive smell, feel, and taste).

THE EXERCISE

Blindfold your partner, and then sit in front of them. Make sure they are comfortable, and then stop speaking. During the course of the exercise, either or both of you may moan, vocalize *ooh* and *ahh*, or giggle. Occasionally an actual word or two may leak out. But this is not a speaking exercise. Talking about each sensation will take both you and your partner away from actually experiencing it.

Concentrate on one sense at a time. I prefer to start with taste because food has taste and texture, as well as temperature and smell—it quickly opens up many senses. Plus, feeding someone is intimate and sweet and generally produces just the right amount of silliness to make the rest of the exercise even more fun. Here's how it works:

Taste. Feed your partner. Actually, don't feed them—tempt them silly. Tease, tease, and tease some more. Run a tasty morsel over their lips and tongue, but don't let them bite it. Allow them to experience the aroma, texture, and temperature of the food, and only then let them have a small bite. Go slowly; don't let them gobble it. This will invite your partner to become the taste of the food or the drink.

Smell. First, smell the item yourself. How strong or subtle is the scent? This will tell you how close to their nose you'll want to put it. Some smells can be overwhelming. Waft the scent by them; don't just shove it under their nose and hold it there. Wait a few seconds between each scent—it gives your partner time to process each one. If your partner prefers, you can offer a sniff of roasted coffee beans between smells to clear the sense memory of the previous smell.

Sound. You can tease with sound, just as you did with taste. Start with subtle, soft little sounds. Use variety. A sound can be near or far, soft or loud, high-pitched or low. Don't forget the infinite variety of the human voice. Whisper a loving word or two into your partner's ear, keeping in mind that this is a sensual delight, not a conversation.

Touch. Touch can be hard or soft, rough or smooth, fast or slow, wet or dry. Whatever you choose, go very slowly and offer only one type of sensation at a time. Remember, you want your partner to experience the sensation so completely that they become the touch.

When you are done, sit silently for a few moments. Then remove your partner's blindfold. Ask your partner to tell you what he or she experienced. Which sensations were particularly nice? Was he or she unable to identify any of the delights? Did any of the sensual delights surprise him or her? How does your partner feel now?

Now switch places; it's your turn to receive.

This exercise can be repeated over and over to refine the quality of the sensations that you and your partner enjoy. If your partner particularly enjoyed some of the softer touches, you can add additional ones, like faux fur or satin sheets. Maybe you discovered that your lover has always been turned on by the smell of urine, semen, or menstrual blood. And who would have guessed that the slow beating of a deep bass drum would drive your partner crazy with desire? When I do this exercise, I am almost always surprised and amazed at how much more there is to experience in a single sensation, particularly in the senses that I do not rely upon primarily. The practice of becoming the taste, touch, sound, and smell of each sensation has taught me how to be more present in each erotic moment. It has also taught me how to make each moment more erotic.

Take what you've discovered in these giving-and-receiving exercises and apply it to all your sexual adventures. Above all, know that you are responsible for your own pleasure. What you ask for, how you receive it, how much you allow, and what you do with it are completely up to you. Your partners are similarly responsible for their own pleasure. When you accept responsibility for your own erotic power and pleasure, here's what happens:

* You stop expecting your partner(s) to be the source of your orgasms.
* You stop pressuring them to give you things you haven't yet learned to accept.
* You stop blaming them for not knowing what you want.
* You learn to articulate to your partner what it is you really want.

Think of yourself as a facilitator of your lover's pleasure, not the source of that pleasure. When two (or more) powerful, responsible, knowledgeable, erotically charged beings come together to share their power in erotic love, there are no limits to where they can go and what they can achieve.

Repeat often: I am the source of my own sexual pleasure.

CHAPTER 14

Rock and Roll

Now it's time to build up some serious orgasmic energy and get it flowing, first within you and then between you and your partner. Commit your full awareness, breath, and body to this portion of your ritual, and you may feel like Shakti and Shiva: pure energy merging with pure consciousness, giving birth to new worlds.

The Heart Connection

Place your right hand over your partner's heart. Your partner places their right hand over your heart. Place your left hand over your partner's right hand (which is on your heart). Your partner places their left hand over your right hand (which is on their heart). See the illustration on the following page.

Breathe together and look into each other's left (or nondominant) eye. Allow a sigh or *ahh* to come out every four or five breaths. Continue for thirty or forty breaths, or until you feel your that your hearts are open and connected.

Now, remove your hand from each other's heart and allow your hands to come together in a prayer position, joining all four hands between you both. Slowly let your hands come apart. Place your hands over your own heart and close your eyes for a few moments. Be aware of where your sexual energy is "hottest" and how it is moving within your body.

VARIATIONS ON THE HEART CONNECTION

You can bring more energy into your heart connection by experimenting with sound and movement.

Do a chakra chant. There are many varieties of chakra chants. One of my favorites is this:

* For the first (root) chakra: lum, lum, lum, lum, lum
* For the second (sex) chakra: vum, vum, vum, vum, vum

* For the third (solar plexus) chakra: rum, rum, rum, rum, rum
* For the fourth (heart) chakra: yum, yum, yum, yum, yum
* For the fifth (throat) chakra: hum, hum, hum, hum, hum
* For the sixth (third eye) and seventh (crown) chakra: om, om, om, om, om

Start on a low pitch for "lum" and raise the pitch for each successive syllable and chakra.

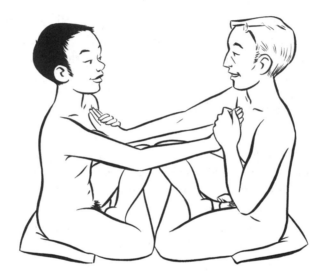

The Heart Connection: Hands to Hearts

Doing a chakra chant with a partner opens, energizes, and harmonizes your energetic body with your partner's.

Add Kegels. When you add Kegels to the Heart Connection, you activate sexual energy deep down in the lower chakras and pump it up to the heart, where it can be shared with your partner.

Rock back and forth. After you have been doing the Heart Connection for a little while, you may find that you have started to rock back and forth. Keep it going! This movement will build your sexual energy and get it flowing between you and you partner. As the rocking becomes faster and more intense, take your hands off each other's hearts and hold them together between you in a prayer position, joining all four hands between you both. As you rock, move your joined hands in circles, sending energy up the front of your body and down the front of your partner's. Then reverse, sending energy up the front of your partner's body and down the front of yours.

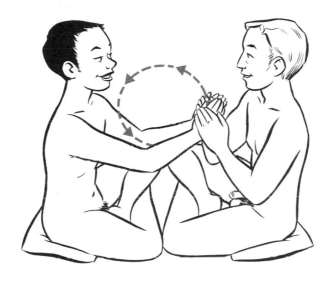

The Heart Connection: Rocking Back and Forth

Warning: Activation of this much heart energy can (and, it is hoped, will) produce a major change of consciousness. Your partner's face may look as if it is changing right in front of you. You may experience massive gigglegasms. You may shed a few tears. It's all good.

Back to Back

Sit back-to-back with your partner, with your backs, heads, and buttocks touching. Breathe. Without using your hands, explore each other's back. Rub, undulate, and caress. Try to feel every contour of your partner's back, buttocks, neck, and head.

Without breaking contact, return to sitting still and upright. With electric vibrators, each of you will now vibrate your own chakras on the front of your body. Start at the root chakra and work your way up your body, chakra by chakra. Make sounds. Allow the vibrations to soften and open each of your chakras. Feel your chakras melt into your partner's.

Spread the Energy Around

Become aware of your entire body by focusing on small areas at a time, or by turning your attention inward and "scanning" your body from toes to head. Are there any areas that are numb or "missing"? Are there any spots that are tense or cramping? Those spots are blocking the flow of your energy like a crimp in a garden hose blocks the flow of water. In order to experience the earth-shaking, consciousness-altering sex you want, you must keep sexual energy moving throughout your entire body. Partners can be enormously helpful with this. Here are some ways to spread energy around:

* Exchange a sensual or erotic massage (see chapters 16 through 18). Build energy in your partner's genitals and spread it up their body and down their arms and legs.
* Kiss up your partner's body from toes to lips. Remember the Resilient Edge of Resistance—if your kisses are too soft or too hard, they may be more ticklish than delicious.
* Flog your partner. Flogging adds intensity, wakes up the system, and releases emotional and physical tension. Flogging does not have to be painful! In fact, some suede floggers are so soft that they would not be capable of causing pain no matter how hard you tried; rather, the receiver experiences a very yummy thud.

Yab Yum/Sitting Position

This classic Tantric position can be done with or without penetration. One partner sits in an easy cross-legged posture or with legs extended in any comfortable position, with a cushion under their tailbone. The other partner sits in their lap, with legs wrapped around their waist and soles of feet touching. For your comfort, be sure to have cushions of various sizes available, for use in different positions.

Both partners place their right hand at the back of their partner's neck and their left hand on their partner's tailbone or lower back. Breathe together and let the energy build.

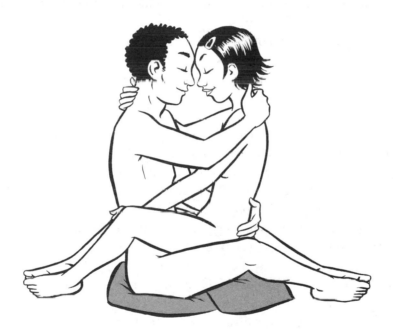

Yab Yum

VARIATIONS ON YAB YUM

Yab Yum is a considerably powerful position. Experiment with these variations, then invent your own.

Leg positions. Unless you want penetration, you do not need to sit in your partner's lap. Even if you do want penetration, you can sit with your legs outstretched over your partner's outstretched legs. You can even sit on chairs. Sit in any position that is comfortable and allows you to get close to your partner. Yab Yum can also be done if one partner is in a wheelchair. However, the partner sitting on top must make sure to move frequently enough to avoid cutting off circulation in their partner's legs.

Breathing in opposition. With mouths touching, as in a kiss, breathe into each other's mouth. One partner breathes in while the other breathes out. This can take a moment to coordinate, but it's worth it. The effect is powerfully trance-inducing. Or, touch your foreheads together, third eye to third eye. Breathe in and out together.

Moving energy up the spine. Draw your left hand up along your partner's spine, from the tailbone to the neck. When your left hand reaches the neck, use your right hand to move the energy up from the neck to the top of the head. Once your hand reaches the top of the head, keep going, moving the energy a foot above the head before placing your hands back in the original position. As you get more and more turned on and active, you may find yourself rocking back and forth passionately. This stroke can be done as quickly and intensely as you like.

Penetration. In the Yab Yum position, you can use a penis, a dildo, a double dildo, or an anal plug for vaginal or anal penetration (see the "Safer Sex" section in chapter 11). Squeeze your PC muscle and visualize a circle of energy enveloping you and your partner. With each inhale and exhale, feel the sexual energy amplifying in you and around you. Imagine the two of you being held in an erotic egg of perfect safety and divine pleasure.

Your partner can turn around so that you can penetrate them from the rear. In this position, you can play with their clitoris or cock. But don't stop there—stimulate all their chakras with a vibrator.

Fuck really fast. Then just stop. Do nothing, and just feel.

Sitting Open-Eyed Clench and Holds

Doing simultaneous open-eyed Clench and Holds with a partner is not only fabulous fun, it's also great practice for keeping your eyes open during all sorts of orgasms.

Sit facing each other. Begin with eye gazing. Breathe together using the Heart Breath or the Circular Breath (see chapter 4). Rock back and forth. Breathe and move to build energy—really go for it. Breathe fuller and faster breaths. When you have built up a lot of energy, take a deep breath and hold it. Stare into each other's eyes and clench your buttocks, abs, and PC muscles.

After about fifteen seconds, let go. Keep your eyes open, and look into your partner's eyes. After a while, either fall backward (away from each other) and close your eyes, or begin breathing again and go for another Clench and Hold—or two or three or more!

Tantric Fucking

There is no such thing as a uniquely Tantric position in which to fuck. If you want a few exciting options, an illustrated copy of the *Kama Sutra* will surely give you some inspiration. The *Kama Sutra* is not actually a Tantric text, although over the centuries, some of the lovemaking positions have been reinterpreted in a Tantric way. It is easy to be intimidated by the number and complexity of sexual poses in the *Kama Sutra*. Many of these positions derive from hatha yoga; and like yoga, positions vary from the simple to the simply outrageous. All of these positions can be reduced to a manageable number of basic postures. The four basic lovemaking positions are

* One lover on top, the other on his/her back
* Both lovers on their sides, facing each other
* One lover with his/her back to the other
* Both lovers in a seated position, usually face to face

Others positions are simply variations on a theme. The most important part of any posture is not how elaborately athletic it is, but how well it facilitates the flow of sexual energy. Key points of connection are the partners' eyes, hands, tongues, breasts, soles of feet, and genitals.

Sex is energy, and energy travels in circuits. When we come together in genital union, our bodies form the most intimate and powerful of energy circuits; sensation is increased and energy is exponentially multiplied.

The art is not in how Tantric a position is,

but how Tantrically you fuck in any position.

Whether you fuck in front, in back, on top, on the bottom, upside down, or right-side up; whether you use dildos, anal plugs, hands, cocks, vaginas, anuses, or mouths, you will be fucking Tantrically if you fuck consciously. What does this mean?

* It means you are breathing.
* It means your attention is focused on your intention. If your intention is to pleasure someone's clitoris, you stay focused on the clitoris and your partner's response to each of your touches.
* It means you are present in the moment and not focusing on some future orgasmic goal.
* It means you are fucking at the Resilient Edge of Resistance—whether your fucking is wild, hard, and loud, or soft, slow, and delicate.

Fuck beyond penetration. Fuck with your hands or your mouth. Combine oral sex with the Erotic Awakening Massage strokes you'll learn in chapters 16 through 18. Combine as many Tantric techniques as you can. Use the power of your imagination. Be creative!

If you have been practicing solo Tantra, you should have a pretty good idea of your most sensitive and receptive erogenous zones. Consciously try positions that will give you the maximum amount of stimulation in those areas. If you love to have your prostate massaged, you could be fucked by a finger or a cock or a dildo or an anal plug. The question is, *how* do you like your prostate massaged? Fast? Slow? With lots of pressure, or with a very light touch? Experiment with your partner until your techniques match your desires.

Mix hard and soft styles in the same position. You can hold your lover down forcefully while you kiss them ever so gently. This is a fast and fabulous way to build a lot of erotic heat.

A last tip: there is a powerful Tantric principle: "three strokes for thirty." It is better to make three delicious strokes precisely at the Resilient Edge of Resistance than thirty strokes that are sloppy and unconscious.

Remember: Three strokes for thirty.

Keep in mind all you have learned about the totality of possibility of orgasm. Your Tantric fucking will likely lead to a physical orgasm or some other orgasmic climax. However, orgasm is not the goal. In Tantra, there is no goal. In this realm, sexual positions and techniques become important not for their ability to produce orgasm, but for their ability to produce prolonged, ever increasing levels of physical delight and consciousness-altering bliss. The climax of this may be huge and thunderingly loud. Or it may be a prolonged ecstatic state accompanied by the sensation of champagne bubbles dancing under your skin. Go totally into the experience of whatever happens. Make no judgments, make no comparisons, and delete your need to understand.

CHAPTER 15

Afterglow

The afterglow is a magical, mystical, fulfilling part of sex that can last longer and be more varied than you might imagine. During the afterglow, some people see colors or visions; some hear music or a universal hum; others feel waves of emotion. Some people feel a deeper intimacy with their partner; others may feel an intimacy with all of creation.

You'll want to stay connected to your partner, but you'll also want to be free to travel on your own postorgasmic journey. These postures will help you make the most of this precious time.

Toes to Third Eye

Lie on your right side. Place your partner's toes at your third eye and hold their feet with your hands. Your partner places your feet on their third eye. Visualize a circuit of energy moving from your third eye to your partner's feet, up their body, through their third eye, into your feet, and up your body. If you like, you can lightly stroke your partner's body with your upper hand.

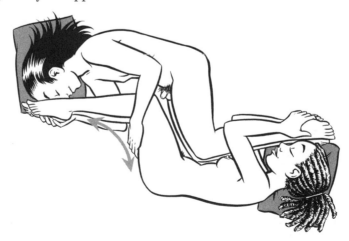

Toes to Third Eye

This is my favorite position for resting after orgasm. I usually do the visualization for the first few breaths, and then I let it go and just meditate. I also love a few minutes of the light stroking. It keeps me aware of my body, allowing me to meditate without drifting off to sleep.

Heart-Foot-Hand

Lie on your backs next to each other with your heads in opposite directions. Your partner should be on your right side. Bend your right leg and place your right foot on your partner's heart chakra. Stretch your left leg out along your partner's right side. Place your right hand on your partner's left foot. Your genitals will be touching. Breathe together. Feel the heart/genital energy circuit and allow your energies to melt and circulate.

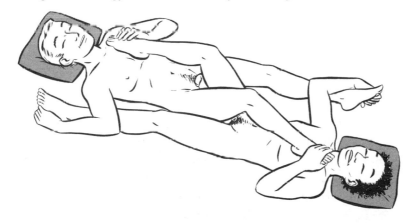

Heart-Foot-Hand

Don't worry if your foot doesn't reach exactly to your partner's heart. It can rest anyplace on the body that feels comfortable. You can even rest it just off your partner's body to the right. The most important thing is that your genitals touch.

This is a peaceful resting posture that you can use at the end of your ritual or between periods of intense sexual activity.

Grounding Hug

The same grounding hug you used in your preparation with your partner is an ideal closing posture as well. It is also a particularly effective technique to use as part of the aftercare in a BDSM scene. It helps bring the submissive partner back to earth without jarring them out of the altered consciousness they've been enjoying. Once again, here's how to give a grounding hug:

Stand with your feet hip-distance apart and your knees slightly bent. Breathe using the Bottom Breath (see chapter 4), bringing your awareness to your root chakra. Imagine that your legs are huge, strong tree roots anchoring you deep into the earth.

Embrace your partner. Place one hand on their lower back, and the other on their upper or middle back. Breathe your belly into their belly. As you hug, imagine that you are grounding your partner in the earth, rooting them the way you are rooted.

Continue breathing together. Feel your partner let go and relax, their center of gravity moving down into their pelvis and legs.

The afterglow does not end when you sit or stand up from your last position. The afterglow from some Tantric rituals can be felt for days. Treat yourself gently. Ease back into your normal life. Pay particular attention to any feelings or inspirations that may arise in the next couple of days. These rituals are powerful energetic events and can provide you with important insights and direction.

You can create an infinite number of rituals using not only these positions and their variations but also a variety of other erotic activities. As you read the following chapters, you'll see the same structure—set the stage, chill out and warm up, come together, rock and roll, and afterglow—applied to other rituals. One of the most remarkable, consciousness-altering uses of this structure is in an erotic massage ritual I call the Erotic Awakening Massage.

CHAPTER 16

The Erotic Awakening Massage: An Introduction

Erotic massage can be a Tantric ritual in itself, and elements of erotic massage can be incorporated into the come together, rock and roll, and afterglow portions of a ritual. Massage is more than foreplay. In fact, I don't even like the word "foreplay." It implies that the only "real" sex is fucking and that everything else is just a warmup to intercourse. In Tantra, virtually everything can be sex. Tantric sex is like a twenty-page menu you'd find in a great diner with all the dishes available as a main course at any time of day. On the Tantric menu, massage—especially erotic massage—is as emotionally, physically, and spiritually satisfying as any great main course fuck.

Choosing the name "Erotic Awakening" for the erotic massage ritual I am about to show you was easy and obvious. In my first experience of receiving this massage, I felt as though I'd awakened from a long sleep. I had found a way to use my sexuality to awaken me to possibilities I had never dreamed of. My subsequent experiences in receiving and giving this massage changed my work; my direction in life; and the way I looked at sex, death, relationships, intimacy, and touch. Not bad for a single technique.

Here are a few of the most meaningful principles I learned:

I learned how to give to someone else without exhausting myself or getting bored. In life as well as sex, I am an overachiever. I would often expend so much energy at the beginning of a lovemaking session that I'd wear myself out just as my partner was warming up. Erotic Awakening Massage provided me with an endless variety of erotic delights to give my partner, which energized me as well. I learned that my partner's body is a wonderfully expressive musical instrument that plays an infinite variety of rhythms. How could I be bored? The effects of this lesson went way beyond sex in that I no longer give so much to other people that I have nothing left for myself.

I learned how to receive while staying conscious and present. It used to be that my mind frequently wandered away during sex. All too often, I would let petty, everyday worries take over my mind; or I would tune out completely and just let someone do me. In order to practice the conscious breath technique that is so much a part of the Erotic Awakening Massage, I had to stay focused on the present.

I learned to ask for what I wanted without feeling guilty. I used to assume that asking for what I liked (especially if I asked for what I really liked) would make my partner unhappy or mad or grossed out. I was afraid that out of love and a desire to please me, my partner would do things they hated. I knew how unhappy and sore and stiff and bored I could get doing something I didn't really want to do, and I sure didn't want to do that to someone I loved! The kind of asking I learned to do during Erotic Awakening Massage gave my partner an opportunity to give me exactly what I like, which in turn made them happy. It also gave them the opportunity to say, "Gee, I'd love to, but my bad back won't let me give you that. What else might you like?" This way I didn't have to feel responsible for their happiness and comfort. Everyone ended up feeling empowered.

I learned how to surrender. Before I practiced Erotic Awakening Massage, I thought of surrender as something I had to do when someone had won some sort of victory over me. On a spiritual level, I thought surrender meant letting go of all control to a higher power—an abstract goal that I had little hope of attaining. On any level, surrender seemed frightening. On the massage table, I learned that surrender is simply a state of vulnerability. I learned not only that vulnerability is safe but also that a vulnerable space is more conducive to maximum growth and pleasure than a well-protected one.

I learned how to give and receive feedback without feeling guilty or taking it personally. When asked to do a simple thing like stroke my lover harder and faster, I used to think "Oh god, I should have known that—I'm such a lousy lover." Nowadays I think, "Oh, I'd love to. Thank you for asking. Is there anything else you'd like?" Talk about a major relief!

I learned that I was capable of sustained heights of pleasure I never knew were possible. We all have our limits. By that I don't just mean how much pain or pleasure we can take. I mean limits on how much we can imagine. If I try to imagine the temperature in the center of the sun or the distance to the farthest star or—in sex—the greatest amount of pleasure I can receive and for how long I can receive it, I will only be able to imagine a portion of what is possible. Anything beyond that point will simply be an abstract mental concept—and a limiting concept at that. Erotic Awakening Massage expanded my awareness of what was possible; it prepared my body to accept levels and stages and lengths of pleasure I could not have imagined.

I even learned how to die. I have explored death more than any other aspect of life on my orgasmic journeys in erotic massage. Far from being depressing or frightening, I have found the spiritual connection between sex and death to be profoundly peaceful and enlightening. I have found more peace and life-guiding revelations in these moments than in any other spiritual or sexual practice. My very first experience receiving erotic massage opened the door to this phenomenon for me.

In 1993, Annie Sprinkle and Joseph Kramer facilitated a workshop called Cosmic Orgasm Awareness Week. There were approximately thirty other participants, many of whom, like me, were coping with AIDS, death, and grief. The highlight and centerpiece of Cosmic Orgasm Awareness Week was giving and receiving what I later developed into the Erotic Awakening Massage. It was designed to raise sexual energy for the healing of whatever needed to be healed—whether or not we knew what that was.

Where Credit Is Due

Joseph Kramer—teacher, sex worker, masseur, therapist, AIDS activist, filmmaker, former Jesuit, and sacred intimate—combined what he'd gleaned from his years of study and practice in Tantra, the Tao, rebirthing, and massage into the genital massage technique on which my Erotic Awakening Massage is based. The original cock strokes were developed by Joseph; the original pussy strokes were developed by Annie Sprinkle and Joseph. (I am proud to say that I was the original crash test dummy for the pussy strokes, which debuted at Cosmic Orgasm Awareness Week.) To order instructional videos for these massages, see the resources section at the end of the book.

After several days of giving and receiving the massage, it was once again my turn to receive. I tried very hard not to have any expectations of what might happen. I tried to stay focused on my breath and on my body. My friend Rod a sensitive and skilled bodyworker, was giving me the massage. After a relaxing and sensual massage, Rod began the erotic strokes—specific strokes on my vulva, clitoris, and G-spot. The sexual energy built up in my body like steam in a pressure cooker. Soon I was approaching orgasm, but not any kind of orgasm I had ever felt before. I began to cry. It was so intense, it felt like if I took one more breath I would fly apart. I took the breath anyway. And everything stopped. There was no light, no sound, no touch—nothing. A blue velvet theatre curtain appeared, and it opened as I approached it. Suddenly I was pulled into a tunnel of blindingly bright light that ended in a vast black nothingness. As my eyes got used to the darkness, I saw stars—thousands of stars. Some of these stars glowed more brightly than others. The brightest star began to speak to me. It was my brother Bill, who had died of AIDS two years before. The bright stars were all my friends who had died. Dozens and dozens of them. I felt myself embraced in one great group hug. "Guys, it is so great to see you all! God, you all look so good! This feels like a big celestial happy hour!"

The feelings of gratitude, fulfillment, and joy at being back together again were overwhelming. I bathed in the love and peace and compassion of my friends. After what seemed like a long time, I felt myself being pulled back and I began to cry again—I wanted to stay. My brother Bill told me what I already knew—that I could not stay.

"You've got too much you've got to do," he said.

"What, what is it I've gotta do? I can't take it back there anymore. It's gotten so bleak and so stodgy and I'm so alone."

"You'll find out," he said. "You'll find out very soon. You're on the right path."

A powerful force pulled me back through the light, and the blue curtain closed when I was on the other side of it. I felt my body around me again. I was still crying, now harder than ever. Then Rod gently draped a sheet over my face and body. It was like being placed in a shroud and dropped into the ground. It was as peaceful and safe as the heavens had been. I felt like I was in the womb. The moment my mind formed this image, I realized I couldn't stay there either. I had to keep going; I was not yet where I was supposed to be. I cried about that, too. Eventually I began to move my body. I became aware of my breath again. Then I felt my body from the inside out. I had arrived at the place I hadn't known how to find. I still didn't know exactly where I was headed, but I knew I had everything I needed to get there: body, breath, and faith. It was all I needed—that, and love. The rest would handle itself.

The Erotic Awakening Massage Has Unlimited Possibilities

It's been years since I started exploring life, sex, and death with the Erotic Awakening Massage, and it still captivates me. One of its most endearing qualities is that it can be adapted for any style or type of erotic relating. This massage is as appropriate for people who have just met as it is for long-term couples looking for new ways to be sexual. It is especially good for lovers looking for new, creative options for safer sex. If you follow the safer sex protocol modeled in these exercises, you can do this massage with no risk of transmitting HIV or other sexually transmitted diseases.

Receiving the Erotic Awakening Massage makes a great alternative for a lover who is paraplegic or quadriplegic, because of the way that the massage combines breath and erotic touch. With the Erotic Awakening Massage, an erotic sensation that begins in a part of the body with no feeling can travel to and be felt in parts of the body that do have feeling.

The Erotic Awakening Massage can be done in a wide variety of styles, from soft and nurturing to hot and hard. Its effects are equally varied. I have seen people laugh with delight from the moment they begin to receive. I have seen people cry. Whatever the style and the immediate response, the Erotic Awakening Massage is capable of remarkable results. It can create greater intimacy between you and a partner. It can take the pressure off sexual performance, and it can take you to new heights and lengths of pleasure. It can release toxins and heal past sexual traumas. The Erotic Awakening Massage can take you deeper into yourself while stretching the limits of who you think you are. It can unite your sexuality and your spirituality. It is a completely new kind of sexual experience.

Sensual Massage

The first part of the Erotic Awakening Massage is sensual massage. Sensual massage is relaxing, opening, enticing, and educing. Eduction is a more generous form of seduction. When we educe, we draw out someone's desire; when we seduce, we persuade them to do what we want to do.

The second part of the Erotic Awakening Massage dances to a strong sexual beat and culminates in waves of pleasure and orgasm. Nothing in this massage is intended to be therapeutic, so it is not your intention to fix anything. You don't need to know deep tissue massage or shiatsu or any other formal massage techniques. You will not be attempting to realign someone's spine or undo the knot in their shoulder. All you need is your breath and your hands.

The two parts of this massage can be done together or separately. You can also take bits and pieces of them and scatter them throughout your other Tantric rituals and sexual play.

Conscious Receiving and Conscious Giving

You need to know only three things to give a great massage: how to breathe, how to touch, and how to ask for feedback. Similarly, you need to know only three things to receive a great massage: how to breathe, how to give feedback, and how to consciously receive. We'll talk about the most challenging of these first: conscious receiving.

Despite the advances women have made in the last century, most women are conditioned to nurture and give to others, and to put themselves last—so much so that many women actually get more pleasure out of giving than receiving. When they make love with someone else, they often deny their own pleasure by thinking they are taking too long to orgasm and that their partner must be getting bored. This massage can teach anyone of any gender how to enjoy the gift of a time and space that is all theirs, in which they might receive all the pleasure and love they can take.

It cannot be overstated that receiving is not a passive activity. As the receiver, you will be participating in this massage; it is not something someone is doing to you. When it is your turn to receive, it's the giver's job to ask what you'd like and how you'd like it, but it's your responsibility to say "a little harder" or "a little softer" or "I'd like something completely different."

When you are the giver, and the receiver gives you feedback—especially unsolicited feedback—you may feel that you have done something wrong. You haven't. Don't take it personally; simply honor their request. (Unless, of course, you are asked to do something you do not wish to do or physically cannot do. In that case, politely ask, "What else would you like?") Say "thank you" in response to feedback. This honors your partner for naming their desire and encourages them to give feedback generously. It also gives you something to say besides "I'm sorry." Sorry for what? Not being able to read their mind? "Thank you" is much more empowering for both giver and receiver.

How to Breathe

The Erotic Awakening Massage is not so much a massage with conscious breathing as it is a conscious breath process with erotic touch. Framing the massage in this way, it's easy to remember that your breathing is the key to your pleasure.

When you are receiving the massage, I recommend you use either the Heart Breath or the Circular Breath (see chapter 4). Breathe in and out of your mouth through slightly parted lips. Keep your neck and jaw relaxed, and your breath easy and unforced. Put your concentration on the inhale; let the exhale just fall out. As the energy builds, your breath will get fuller and faster. That's perfect. Just make sure you're not forcing it.

When you are giving the massage, it is equally important that you keep your breath conscious. I recommend using the Circular Breath. Also, try to match your breath to your partner's. It will help you stay at their Resilient Edge of Resistance.

Whole-Hand Touching

The secret of great touch is whole-hand touching. When you touch with your whole hand, it feels like an embrace, as if the touch is actually coming straight from your heart. Many people touch less with their hands and more with their fingertips. This can feel more like poking. Occasional fingertip stroking can be delicious, but massage with fingertips is often symptomatic of fearful touch and is more likely to produce a tickle response. A light touch is not the same thing as a tentative touch. A light touch is the conscious use of less pressure; it is intentionally light, not tentatively light.

Let's try it. First, find the little indentation in the middle of your palm. That's the heart of your palm. Now touch your thigh or arm, making contact with the heart of the palm first, and then letting the rest of your hand relax around it. That's whole-hand touching. Whole-hand touching massages the hands of the giver as well as the body of the receiver—a lovely bonus.

Gliding. The first stroke we'll do with whole-hand touching is called *gliding.* Try it on your own body. Place your hands on your lower leg, hearts of palms first. Let the fingers just relax around the curves of your leg. Allow your hands to conform to the contours of your ankle and calf. Then slowly pull your hands toward you, allowing your fingers to trail behind. Follow the shapes of the muscles and bones underneath the skin. When you are massaging someone else, you can glide from your partner's shoulder all the way down their back, over their buttocks, down their leg to their foot, and back again with one long gliding stroke. Don't lift your hands. Go *slowly.* I have never heard anyone complain that a massage was done too slowly. The secret to gliding is to keep your hands relaxed and pull them toward you; don't push them away from you.

Kneading. This is a great complementary stroke to use with gliding. Using your whole hand, press into the muscle, and then suck the flesh into your palm, the way a kitten kneads its mother's belly to get the milk to flow. Knead with your palm, and let your fingers follow. This stroke can feel embracing and relaxing or deep and stimulating, depending on your intention. Stay at your partner's Resilient Edge of Resistance.

Vibrations. Vibrations are a great way to get muscles to relax. Vibrations can go very deep, but they are not invasive. Try it on your thigh. Place your hands, palms first, on either side of your thigh. Let your fingers relax. With alternating side-to-side motion of your hands, begin a rather fast vibration of your thigh muscles. Feel the resilience in the muscles and skin. Adjust the speed of your vibrations until you feel a natural wave in the muscles of your thigh. If a muscle is tense, it will take faster vibrations to make that wave. As the muscle relaxes, you can slow down. Ideally, you want to use a vibration that's as effortless and as slow as possible. Vibrations feel particularly great on the buttocks. Try vibrating both cheeks in sync with each other, then out of sync, then in sync again. It feels great, and it's silly fun, too.

Lifting and holding. Lifting and holding an arm or a leg can be a lovely way to release tension and practice trust. When you want to move an arm or a leg, be sure to support the joints, holding them with the same whole-hand touch you've been using for the other strokes. You can gently pull a limb away from the body and then replace it. Remember, this is not therapeutic massage. Your intention is to help your partner relax and drop into their body.

The Resilient Edge of Resistance. A sensual massage should not be so soft that it tickles your partner or puts them to sleep. Keep in mind the Resilient Edge of Resistance. Go as deep as you can while still finding resilience. If a muscle becomes rigid, you've gone too far. If the muscle feels flaccid, you haven't gone far enough. Play with the elasticity of the flesh and find the edge where there is both resistance and resilience. That's where your touch will be the most aware, awake, and pleasurable.

How do you know you're at the Resilient Edge of Resistance?

You push and the body pushes back just a little.

Stillness. There is another extremely powerful stroke that is all too often ignored in nearly every type of massage. That stroke is stillness. Do not make the common mistake of thinking that giving a massage means being in constant motion. One of the most sensuous, healing, and powerful ways of being with someone is simply to hold them. Embrace with your hands; with the hearts of your palms. Breathe.

This is all you need to know about touch to give a luxurious, muscle-melting massage. Naturally, all the strokes can be combined in any manner. Just remember, your best instructors are your breath, your intuition, and your partner. Follow your instincts and ask, ask, ask for feedback.

Gender and the Erotic Awakening Massage

The Erotic Awakening Massage was originally divided into two types: one for men and one for women. That was in the days when we thought of gender—even biological gender—as either/or. Early on in my practice with these massages, I began to notice that this arbitrary division based on genital innies and outies was much too limiting. There was simply too much crossover.

My understanding of the "more than two" school of sex and gender began when a brave transperson—self-identified "spansexual" norrie m⊕y welby—asked if she could attend my Yoni Massage workshop in Sydney. (Yoni—Sanskrit for vagina—Massage was the name for an earlier version of the Erotic Awakening Massage.) I asked norrie if she had a yoni; norrie said yes. I said, "Then please do join us." That weekend, as I was explaining the massage strokes for the G-spot, I asked norrie if she had a G-spot. She said she didn't know. norrie was born a boy, with a penis and testicles. norrie later had gender reassignment surgery, which reshaped the penis and testicles into a vagina and clitoris. Although norrie's surgery was intended to "make her a woman," she now lives as both/neither and/nor male/female. norrie knew that she still had a prostate gland and that P-spot stimulation felt good. When norrie was male, the only way to reach his P-spot was through his anus. Now that norrie had a vagina, her P-spot could also be stimulated by pressing against the back wall of her vagina.

In the course of the Erotic Awakening Massage, norrie discovered that she also had a G-spot. What's more, G-spot massage strokes on her new yoni felt as good as the P-spot strokes. Now the other women in the workshop wanted to try the P-spot strokes—which were, after all, simply the G-spot strokes done on the opposite wall of the vagina. And guess what? More than half the women reported that the P-spot strokes felt great. Although the genetic women did not have a prostate and norrie did not have a urethral sponge, there was something present in both cases that liked being stimulated.

This kind of genital gender-bending became more and more common as I relaxed and reframed my notion of which strokes were for pussies and which were for cocks. I invite you to relax your own gendered notions of genitalia. For the sake of readability and ease in communicating the strokes, I will be a bit less postmodern. In the next two chapters, I will describe one massage for people with vulvas and vaginas (chapter 17), and one for people with penises and testicles (chapter 18). I will use the pronoun *she* to refer to a person with a pussy, and the pronoun *he* to refer to a person with a cock. I do not mean to offend or exclude the hunky gentlemen I know with vaginas or the many gorgeous ladies with penises. And for all of you with something in between or something other than a pussy or a cock, I invite you to mix and match. (I do, even when I am playing with more traditional genitals.) Take what works for you from either or both massages and discard the rest.

If you have a vulva and vagina, I would suggest you start with the massage for people with pussies. If you have a cock, start with the massage for people with penises. Both massages begin with sensuous touch, but following that, they are paced quite differently. The massage for people with pussies starts slowly and builds progressively, as if climbing an incline toward high-energy orgasm. The massage for people with penises, while intended to build energy, is also designed to avoid ejaculation, so it is much more of a roller-coaster ride of fast, energizing strokes alternating with slow, relaxing strokes.

Orgasm and the Erotic Awakening Massage

The Erotic Awakening Massage will provide you with new and expanded orgasmic experiences, both genital and energetic. The Erotic Awakening Massage for people with pussies often produces multiple physical orgasms. The Erotic Awakening Massage for people with penises can also provide multiple orgasms, so long as the person with a penis does not ejaculate. (In fact, the Erotic Awakening Massage for people with penises is ideal practice for those eager to learn the art of male multiple orgasm.) The simple fact is that women (or those with estrogen-based bodies) can have multiple orgasms—with or without ejaculation—with little loss of sexual energy. Men (or those with testosterone-based bodies who ejaculate through their penises) suffer a near-total loss of sexual energy after ejaculation. Therefore, in order to experience the extended and expanded pleasure states available in prolonged arousal, ejaculation is to be avoided.

Both versions of the Erotic Awakening Massage end with the Clench and Hold energy orgasm technique. When we practiced the Clench and Hold earlier (see chapter 9) we used breath to charge the body. In the Erotic Awakening Massage, in addition to your breath, you will also be charging your body with movement, sound, and genital massage. The exponential effect of this combination greatly enhances the orgasmic and mystical potential of the Clench and Hold.

Important reminder: Lungs are genderless; the most important

part of the Erotic Awakening Massage is the conscious breathing.

Over the course of the past decade, I have done this massage in countless workshops, demonstrations, and private sessions. The more I do it, the less I know. That is why I am still so passionate about it. I invite you to become as clueless as I am. After you've become familiar with the basics of the Erotic Awakening Massage, get creative! Make it your own. Create new strokes, new ways of breathing, and new forms of sensuous touch; and put it all together at the pace that works for you. Oh—one more note before we begin. Most of the strokes have short, humorous names to make it easy for you to remember them and ask for them. Ask and it shall be given, and it shall be delightful.

CHAPTER 17

The Erotic Awakening Massage for People with Pussies

This version of the Erotic Awakening Massage has the same structure as any other Tantric ritual, with one slight modification. First, you'll set the stage for your massage. Next, instead of chilling out and warming up, you'll come together with your partner so that you can both share your thoughts or feelings that need to be spoken before the massage actually begins. The chill out and warm up portion of the ritual is a luxurious sensual massage followed by the first of the genital strokes. This soon intensifies into rock and roll as the genital strokes become more specifically arousing. Finally, following a Clench and Hold, the receiver enters a long afterglow filled with endless possibilities.

Setting Up

Start by creating a serene space for your massage by choosing a comfortably warm room with soft lighting, lots of fresh air, and music with a gentle, steady rhythm. You certainly can do the massage without music, but I find that the right music helps both receiver and giver to maintain conscious breathing. Plus, this massage is such a great dance, it's a shame to do it without music.

Put a towel and a sheet on your massage table. If you don't have a massage table, you can use another kind of table or the floor. Although it may seem logical to use a bed, beds are usually at an uncomfortable height for the person who is giving the massage. It's important for both of you to be comfortable at all times. As the giver, you don't want a sore back at the end of your partner's pleasure.

If you are the giver, make sure your fingernails are not too long or too sharp. Trim any ragged edges. Check your hands for any calluses and smooth them down with a pumice stone.

Next, gather the things you'll need: latex or vinyl gloves, condoms, lube, and massage oil or cornstarch (also known as corn flour). Cornstarch? Yes. Instead of oil, you might like the feel of cornstarch on your skin. It's like getting a massage with powdered silk. It's hypoallergenic and it's easy to clean up—just shake it out or vacuum it up.

Connecting

When you're set up and ready to begin, take a moment to connect with your massage partner. You might sit face to face and breathe together as you gaze into each other's eyes. Find that place of connection between the two of you that needs no words—that place of mirroring where you can see the best of yourself in her and her best in you. Try to look beyond the physical to actually see her spirit.

This is a time for speaking. Tell each other how you are feeling. Let your partner know any physical or medical limitations you may have. If you are receiving, tell your partner if there are any places on your body that are especially tense. Do you have a special request? Perhaps there is something you want to heal or create in your life. You can make that desire the focus of the energy raised in this massage by making a dedication (see chapter 22 for more on dedicating sexual energy). If you're the giver, you may have intentions and needs to express as well. Now is the time to speak these. You are partners in this experience.

Starting with a Sensual Massage

The receiver lies on the table or floor, face down. The giver might begin the sensual massage with the touch of something other than a hand. Try an ostrich feather or a silk scarf. Your intention is to help your partner relax and come to a deeper awareness of her body. So alternate elegant, relaxing strokes with different types of touch that are a bit more stimulating. You could use a loofah sponge (mild) or a cat-o'-nine-tails (wild). (See the "Props: Mild to Wild" chart in chapter 11 for other ideas.) When you're both ready to move on, lovingly apply cornstarch or massage oil. Give her a sensual massage using the whole-hand touching strokes you learned earlier.

Remember her hands, her feet, and her head. We carry so much tension in these places. Massage her feet; gently pull her toes. On your way up to the top of her head, do the same for her hands. Then massage her scalp.

Gently massage her breasts with whole-hand circular glides. This helps open her heart center. Spread the heart energy down her arms and then down her torso.

ARE YOU BREATHING?

Take a moment to make sure you are both breathing consciously. You can help the woman receiving the massage to keep breathing by staying conscious of your own breathing. The idea is not to control her breathing, but to set up a rhythm with her. When the two of you are breathing in a rhythm and at a pace that's comfortable for you both, you've established another level of connection. The rhythm of the music can help.

WAKING UP THE NEIGHBORHOOD

Now that your partner has relaxed and dropped into her body, it's time to begin building some erotic energy.

Over Eggs Easy. Glide your palms in circles on her abdomen, in the area where her ovaries are, or were, or would have been. Not all people with pussies have ovaries or uteruses. Whatever lies beneath the surface, these are still important sexual energy centers. Alternate circles with stillness. Remember the Resilient Edge of Resistance, and both you and your partner will stay relaxed and energized.

The Womb Warmer. Glide your palms in circles on her abdomen, in the area where her uterus is, or was, or would have been. Don't be afraid to use some pressure—it can feel really good on an exhale. But be sensitive, especially if the woman is menstruating. Look for feedback in how she is responding to your touch, and when in doubt, ask. Alternate circles with stillness.

The Heart-Womb Palm Rest. Rest one hand over her womb, and the other over her heart. Breathe with her. This stroke connects her energized womb with her heart.

Sensual Glove Strokes. Familiarize your partner with the feel of latex or vinyl. Dance a pair of gloves gently over her skin; or try a more energizing stroke—a fast, circular slapping motion up and down her body. A flogging with gloves is guaranteed to produce lots of energy and lots of laughs. It makes a lot of noise and doesn't hurt at all. Put on the gloves and keep them on until the end of the massage. Place your hands on her womb and heart. Turn the hand on her womb toward her feet and move it over her pubic mound and genitals, and you're ready to begin the next stroke.

The Heart-Pussy Palm Rest. Rest one hand over her genitals, and the other hand over her heart. You are connecting heart energy and sexual energy. Just be still and be there.

The Outer Labia Acupress. With the sides of your forefingers of both hands, press where the outer labia meet the thighs. This stroke helps your partner open herself to pleasure. Press, release, press, release.

The Pubic Hair Pull. Grab fingerfuls of her pubic hair and lift. Don't yank or jerk. Don't tug on one hair at a time. Do scratch vigorously. Knead the pubic mound. This stroke feels great if it's used sparingly, but it can get annoying if you overdo it. Stay conscious and in touch with each other so you'll know the difference.

ARE WE BREATHING?

As giver, take another moment to make sure you are breathing consciously. Take a long, full, deep, audible breath. This will encourage your partner to breathe. There are numerous effective ways to encourage breathing throughout the course of the massage. Some of my favorite breath-coaching cheers include: "Wouldn't a nice full breath feel good right now?" or "There's so much nice, fresh air in the room; it's a shame we're not using more of it." Some people might prefer the sassier "If you don't breathe, I'll turn off the vibrator," or "Okay, don't breathe—see if I care! " That one is most effective when followed by an evil laugh. It's all a matter of style.

The Vulva

Help your partner find a comfortable position. Her legs can be stretched out along the length of the table; or her knees can be raised, with her feet flat on the table. She can also put the bottoms of her feet together, with her knees apart. Use pillows under her knees for extra support.

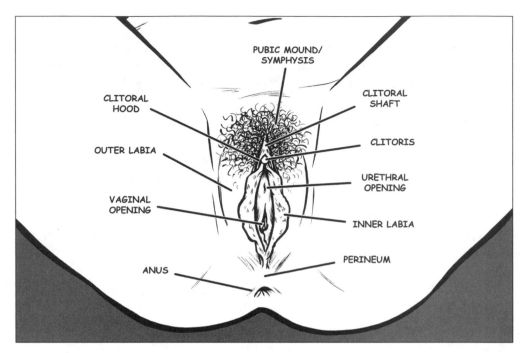

The Vulva

Vibrate That Vulva. Place your entire hand over her vulva. Hold and vibrate.

Pussy Petting. Lubricate your hands. Ask if she'd like the lube warmed or cool. To warm the lube, pour a generous amount onto one palm and hold your hands together for a few moments. Pet her pussy with long, slow strokes from bottom to top, and then top to bottom. (Avoid the anus. You don't want to introduce any bacteria from her anus into her vagina. It can cause a nasty infection.)

The Three-Finger Pussy Pet. Using your three longest fingers, glide the middle finger between the two inner labia as the other two fingers slide along the space between the inner and outer labia on each side. You can hold the vulva open with your other hand, if that makes it easier.

The Outer/Inner Labia Massage. Hold each of her labia between your thumb and fingertips and lovingly massage each of the outer labia, and then each of the inner labia. Be very specific and go slowly. Labia sizes will vary widely. Whatever you discover is both normal and unique.

Tour de France. With one hand, gently pull the pubic mound up toward her belly to open the vulva. With the forefinger of your other hand, trace a circle between inner and outer labia from the perineum to above the clitoris and back to the perineum. For extra yum, add a little loop around the clitoris.

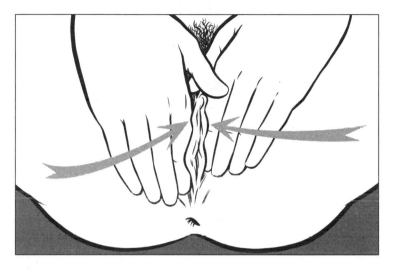

The Mushy Puss

The Mushy Puss. Place your flattened hands on either side of the vulva and smoosh the labia together with the sides of your index fingers. Use a little pressure, because the clitoris is there in between getting a nice little stroke.

Divine Drumming. Tap the inner thighs and vulva with your flat hand, as if playing a drum. Ask for her feedback—harder? Softer? A fast rhythm? Slow, single drumbeats? Be sensitive with this one. Some women like quite intense drumming; others might not like it as hard. A single drumbeat can send a charge of energy all the way to the top of her head. Receiver, don't wait to be asked for feedback; ask for what you want. Giver, remember to say "thank you" whenever she names her desire.

The Breath of Spring. Gently part her labia and blow air on them. Get closer and it's a warm wind; stand back and it's a cool breeze.

Time for a breathing check:

How is she doing? How are you doing?

The Clitoris

Open the labia and pull back the clitoral hood, revealing the clit. Some clits are shy and small. Others are bold and big. All clits are highly sensitive. Don't just grope around blindly! If you lose sight or feel of the clit (or G-spot or labia or anything else), stop, find it, and then proceed. That's the difference between conscious touch and unsatisfying groping. Keep your attention where your intention is.

Flutterby. Gently touch and tickle her clitoris. Use an intentional but very light touch. Think of a butterfly's wings. This touch can be slow or rapid. Ask which she prefers.

Rock around the Clit Clock. This stroke is a huge favorite. Pretend that the clit is the center of a clock. With your forefinger, make tiny circles immediately to the side of the clit, stopping at the location of each "hour." Tell her what "time" it is at each stroke, and ask which she likes best. Every person with a pussy will have a favorite hour. Two o'clock is very popular. Six o'clock is popular as well.

Pinch and Pull. Using plenty of lube, try to pinch and pull the clit. (If you can actually pinch and pull it, you are not using enough lube!) You will be stroking down the clitoral hood, with the clitoral shaft underneath it. It feels amazing.

As She Likes It. Any requests? There's a good reason why all the strokes have fun, easy-to-remember names. It's so you can ask for what you want easily. Ask her how she would like her clit massaged. She can ask you to repeat a stroke, or she may make up a new one!

Spreading the Energy Around

Involve her whole body. Beginning with any of the pussy strokes you've just learned, move on to spread the energy down her thighs and legs and up her body to her heart, her third eye, and the top of her head. Use your sensual massage strokes, particularly glides and kneading. Do this frequently and at any time during the massage. Keep returning to her vulva to reenergize.

Intravaginal Massage

It is always important to ask the receiver what she wants and enjoys, but never more important than now. Not every person with a pussy likes to be penetrated. And those women who do like to be penetrated deserve the courtesy of being asked. So this is the time to ask. If she says yes, enter her gently and slowly. If she is menstruating, you may need to remove a tampon. Remind her to breathe and relax; then gently remove the tampon, wrap it in a paper towel, and throw it away.

One Finger. Use lots of lube. Very slowly, insert your well-lubed forefinger. (You did trim your fingernails, right?) Don't do anything once you are inside, just be there. This is a wonderful time to breathe together and bring energy up to her heart.

Two Fingers. Ask if she would like another finger. If she says yes, enter her with a second finger. *Slowly* so that she has time to tell you to stop or slow down when she has had enough. Going slowly can also be delicious for the giver. Go completely into the experience of feeling what you're touching.

The Four Directions. With one or two fingers inside her vagina, stroke or press firmly upward (toward the ceiling). Turn your hand 90 degrees clockwise and press to one side. Turn your hand 90 degrees clockwise again and press downward (toward the floor). Turn your hand 90 degrees clockwise once more and press to the other side. Repeat. Be aware of how much pressure you're using. Firm pressure may feel yummy, but start gently.

The Goddess Spot (a.k.a. the G-Spot). Locate and massage the entire urethral sponge with one or two fingers. The G-spot—the spot of greatest sensitivity—is located on the urethral sponge. The urethral sponge is the tissue of the upper (toward the ceiling) wall of the vagina. The texture of the G-spot is different from that of surrounding vaginal walls, which is smooth. The G-spot ranges in size from a half-inch to two inches in diameter, depending upon the woman and how stimulated she is. It has a rougher, sometimes ribbed or nubbly, texture.

Enter her with one finger and make a "come hither" gesture with it. You will probably know when you find it by her reaction. But you can only be sure by asking her, so communication is key. Stimulating the G-spot tends to produce a jolting or electrically charged feeling. She may suddenly feel as though she has to pee. Start gently on the G-spot, but if you are having trouble finding it, you can try reaching in a little further and pressing a bit more firmly.

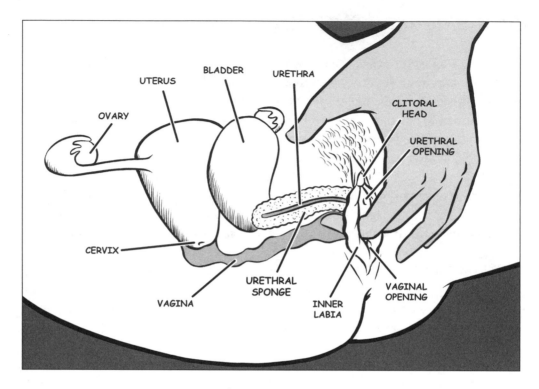

The G-Spot

The Doorbell. Press firmly on her G-spot, as if ringing a doorbell. Press, release, press, release . . .

G-Spot Massage. Apply steady pressure, circling around her G-spot in both directions. Stroke back and forth. Add clitoral stimulation with your other hand. Alternate between G-spot stimulation and clitoral stimulation; try ten seconds of each. Invite her to add Kegels. Kegels increase sexual energy and move it up the body.

Stop!

As the energy starts to build, it is even more important for you as the giver to remember to stop and center yourself and breathe with your partner for a moment. Just stop. Remember the power of stillness. These moments give the receiver time to integrate the energy and prepare her to move to even higher states of erotic charging.

The Cervix. The cervix is the narrow outer end of the uterus, located at the upper rear of the vagina. Some women who have a cervix like to have it pushed against. But even if a person with a pussy does not have a cervix, she may still like a thrusting stroke. Ask before you thrust. Go easier during menstruation.

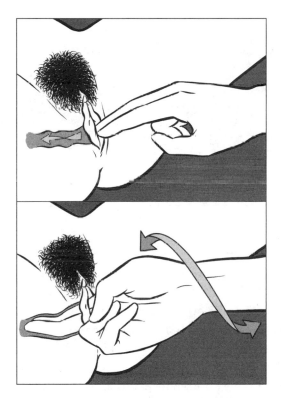

Twist and Shout

Twist and Shout. Using one, two, or three fingers, penetrate in and out while twisting at the wrist. Your knuckles will roll past her G-spot. Twist and shout is a thrusting stroke, and thrusting strokes increase energy. Remind her about Kegels—they make it even more energizing. If she is breathing and moving her pelvis, she may be meeting your hand halfway; you won't have to do much except twist your hand and meet her.

The Healing Thrust. This is a perfect stroke to alternate with twist and shout. It is the same thrust, without the twist. She may like this thrust slow, deep, and hard, or fast and shallow. Ask her to be specific. Many women have experienced penetration they felt they had no control over or penetration they did not want. This conscious penetration, which she can control with her feedback, may be empowering and healing, or just plain feel wonderful. Be sure to encourage her to breathe and relax.

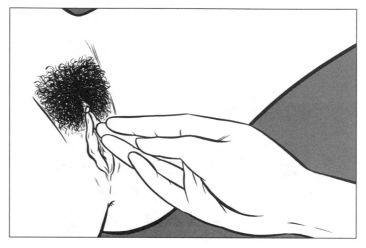

Filled with Love

Filled with Love (a.k.a. fisting). Some people with pussies might enjoy having a whole fist inside their vagina. Make sure she is very relaxed and breathing deeply. Start with two fingers, and then add a third. Tuck your thumb under all four fingers and curl your fingers inward. This stroke is not a thrusting motion; it's a twist. You'll know pretty quickly whether your hand will slide in past your knuckles or not. If it doesn't, stop. If it does, stop when you are inside. Just stop and be still. Bring your awareness to your breath. Appreciate that feeling of going back to the womb. This stroke works wonders to relax the whole pelvis and builds a lot of life/sex energy. Try it with your other hand under her tailbone, or while massaging her abdomen with your other hand.

Stillness. Hold completely still while your hand or fingers are inside her vagina. Don't move; just be there; meditate.

Rock and Roll

This section of the massage uses a vibrator. A battery-operated vibrator is neither strong nor subtle. Rechargeable vibrators may lose their charge before you are finished. A vibrator that plugs into the wall is the way to go. To maintain safer-sex protocol, put a large latex glove over the head of a large vibrator, and plastic wrap on the handle. You can use condoms for wand-type vibrators; roll the condom down the shaft.

Think of the vibrator as an extension of your hands. In all the following strokes, feel for that Resilient Edge of Resistance. Too much pressure with the vibrator will hurt, but too little feels annoying.

Start at the bottoms of her feet, and move up her legs. Then vibrate her chakras. At the first chakra, place your hand between the vibrator and her pussy. Then move up to her belly, her solar plexus, then her heart and nipples. Anytime you are using the vibrator over a bony area, put your hand between the vibrator and her body. This is especially important around the throat. (You may want to vibrate the throat chakra by placing the vibrator—at slow speed—at the back of her neck.) Vibrate the center of her forehead and the top of her head.

Now vibrate her inner thighs and around her outer labia to get her used to the sensation of the vibrator and to tease her unmercifully.

Vibrate around the Clit Clock. Place the vibrator on top of your lubricated forefinger and place your finger at twelve, three, six, and nine o'clock.

Vibrate the Clitoris. Some women don't like the vibrator directly on the clitoris. You can use a finger beneath the vibrator; or you can apply the vibrator to one side of her clit. Use enough lube to make sure the vibrator glides easily.

The Vibrating Doorbell. Press, release, press, release with the vibrator on her vulva and clitoris.

Vibrate the Vaginal Opening. Place the head of the vibrator at the vaginal opening.

As She Likes It. Ask her how and where she'd like her vibrations.

Freestyle. By this time, the energy will probably be rocketing along nicely. Remind her to breathe. Use whole-hand strokes to spread the energy around her body, and just try to keep up with her. This section of the massage can get loud and wild and crazy. (Don't you just love that?) She may have an orgasm, or several; she may not. There is no goal. You are using breath and erotic energy in whatever form it chooses to take to charge of the body. Let whatever happens happen. Simply focus on building and circulating as much sexual energy as possible.

The Clench and Hold

When her body is fully charged with breath and sexual energy, it's time for the Clench and Hold. Invite her to take about thirty fast, full breaths and then three big, deep breaths. She holds the third deep breath and tenses every muscle in her body, especially her buttocks and abdomen.

Remember, there are a number of ways to do this clench. She can

* Press downward onto the massage table or floor with her hands and shoulders, head and butt, and legs and feet
* Extend her body outward as far as it can go, reaching for the opposite walls with her feet and her hands
* Pull in toward the center of her body as hard as she can, first clenching her abdominal muscles, and then pulling the rest of her body in toward her abs

When she takes the third deep breath, remove your hands and the vibrator. Count silently to fifteen, and then tell her to let go and relax.

Now What?

This is the most profound portion of the massage, for both giver and receiver. If you have been giving the massage, sit or stand nearby quietly and breathe. Don't talk to your partner or touch her. Just let her be for fifteen to thirty minutes. Notice how you are feeling. Although you will want to keep some of your awareness on your partner, use this time for yourself as well. What was your experience? Although there is no goal in this massage, the emphasis is on going into a new place of meditation and relaxation within ourselves, and this can be true for the giver as well as the receiver.

If the receiver indicates that she wants to be covered up, gently fold the sheet around her. She may want her face covered. For some women, this feels like being held safely in the arms of mother earth; for others it may feel like a tomb. Everyone's experience of this process will be different. There is no right or wrong way to feel. Some women who receive this massage may not feel very much the first time. Some may need more time to work with the conscious breath techniques and practice receiving in order to relax and receive pleasure. Some women, especially those who have been sexually abused, may cry or feel angry or numb. Allow whatever needs to happen to happen. She may laugh or cry or yell, or lie there so still and peacefully that she looks as if she has died. Resist the temptation to hug her or comfort her unless she specifically asks you to.

When she indicates that she is ready to move, help her roll onto her side, and eventually to sit up. Remember that you have been spreading her energy and her juices around her body. To maintain safer-sex protocol, do not touch her until she has had a shower or unless you are still wearing (or have put on a fresh pair of) gloves. If you want to hug as she gets off the table, make sure her sheet is between you.

This erotic massage is a healing and clearing process. Many women report feeling more sensitive for a few days after receiving this massage. Some feel great, some cry more easily, some notice that they feel all their emotions more intensely, and some feel relaxed and energized. Be gentle with her and be gentle with yourself.

You have just experienced a new and powerful way of relating erotically: an experience of pure giving and pure receiving. Take some time to express gratitude to your partner for sharing this experience with you, and communicate something of what the experience was like for you. Try to avoid slipping back into old patterns. If you were the one receiving, don't immediately start thinking of what you can do for your partner. If you were the one giving, don't quiz your partner on how you could have done it better. Speak from your heart. Use the time and your experience to deepen and expand your own lives and to grow in your relating with each other.

CHAPTER 18

The Erotic Awakening Massage for People with Penises

The Erotic Awakening Massage for people with penises begins much like the massage for people with pussies. After all, both pussies and penises are connected to bodies, minds, and spirits, all of which get attended to in the course of this massage. But as explained in chapter 16, this version of the massage is designed to prevent ejaculation, creating deeper (and even multiple) orgasms.

If you haven't already, please read the sections called "Setting Up" and "Connecting" in chapter 17. Prepare a serene space with soft lighting, fresh air, and nice music. Gather the things you'll need: latex or vinyl gloves, condoms, lube, and massage oil or cornstarch. Connect with each other before you begin to touch. You can ask yourself and each other, "What wants to be spoken now so that we can both surrender to the massage when the touching begins?"

Here is a special note for the person receiving: Please remember that, although it is the job of the person giving the massage to ask what you would like and how you would like it, it is also your job to tell them. Receiving is not a passive activity. This massage is a process you are participating in, not something someone is doing to you. It is your responsibility to say "a little harder," "a little softer," "a little more to the right," and of course, "ooh, that's nice." And givers, sometimes when the receiver says "not so hard" or "a little to the left," you may think, "Oh, I have done something wrong." No, you haven't. Don't take it personally; simply do what they ask. In fact, it's nice to say "thank you" whenever you get feedback. The thank-you honors the receiver for naming his desire.

Although this erotic massage will focus on his cock, you will want to remember to spread his sexual energy all throughout his body and, in particular, you will want to open the energy channel between his cock and his heart. The natural heart/cock connection is often damaged in the process of growing up male in the Western world, where men are encouraged to act more from the first and second chakras than the heart chakra. Only in the last couple of decades has the archetype of the sensitive New Age guy become acceptable, and even then, just barely. This massage can be a great healer of the heart/cock schism.

The style of this erotic massage for people with penises is to build up energy in the cock with specific cock strokes and then distribute that energy throughout the body. From the cock, we will bring energy into the belly and the heart and then distribute it from these centers into the arms and legs. By bringing sexual energy away from the cock and into the rest of the body, we charge the entire body with sexual energy while avoiding ejaculation. Remember, we are not trying to avoid orgasm—only ejaculation, which would deplete the sexual energy.

The strokes we will use to concentrate and distribute the energy are circles and U-shaped strokes. A *U* is a glide with your palm from the belly or heart or perineum out to both arms or both legs. For example, from the heart, you glide from the nipple down to the knee, back up to the same nipple, over to the other nipple, and then down to the other knee. From the belly or perineum, it's the same: glide from the belly or perineum to the knee, back up to where you began, and then down to the other knee. Circles concentrate energy; *U*s distribute them. Use a circular stroke on the belly or heart or perineum to concentrate sexual energy in those areas, and then use a *U* to distribute that energy further.

Gather your latex gloves and grab some lube (or if he prefers massage oil, grab your vinyl gloves), and let's get started.

Starting with a Sensual Massage

Invite your person with a penis to lie on his back. Invite him (or order him, if that's the style you've both agreed upon) to breathe.

Begin with a sensual massage. Try tantalizing him with a feather or a scarf. One touch that many men find deliciously awakening is a light brushing over the top of any body hair they may have. When you are ready to begin the sensual massage strokes, you can use cornstarch, oil, or just your bare hands. You do not need to put on your gloves until you are about to touch his cock. Take your time with the sensual massage. The key to all erotic massage is relaxation. It may sound strange to hear that you want your partner to be totally relaxed if you want to be sexual with them, but it's true. After he is completely relaxed, you can add any amount of conscious tension you want. This is much better for eroticism than being driven or blocked by the many little unconscious tensions we all carry around most of the time.

Help your partner maintain an even, conscious breath by breathing evenly and consciously yourself. Matching your breath to your partner's is a surefire way to instant intimacy. After you have relaxed his body, you can start to wake up the genital area. Many men focus most of their awareness on the glans—the head of the penis. Waking up the area around the penis opens the energetic pathways between the cock and the rest of the body.

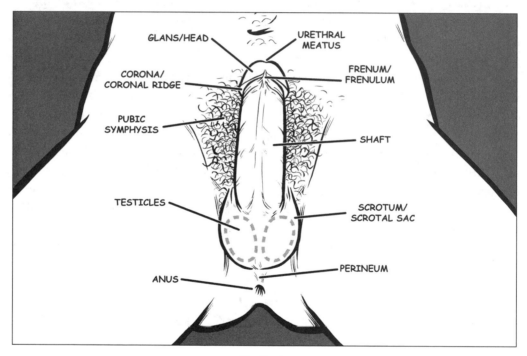

The Penis

You can tug on his pubic hair, just not one hair at a time! Grab fingerfuls of it and lift. You can scratch vigorously in his pubic hair. Knead the whole pubic symphysis—the flesh over the pubic bone. Gently take the skin between your thumb and forefinger and knead it.

Now tickle or gently tug on the hair of the scrotum. If the skin of the scrotum is fairly loose, you can knead it. Don't knead the testicles, just the scrotal skin. Knead it between your finger and thumb, stretching it until you find the Resilient Edge of Resistance—that is, until you feel it start to pull back.

The Cock Strokes

Now it's time to put on your gloves and begin the cock strokes.

Cock Shiatsu. This is a great wake-up stroke. Grasp the head of his cock and stretch it to its full length. Cocks are elastic—they stretch quite easily. Hold his cock in the stretched position between finger and thumb. Using your other hand, squeeze a finger width at a time from base to glans and back. You can work quite deeply. You can do this laterally (from the sides) and then along the top and bottom (dorsal and ventral). This is a stroke to awaken the entire shaft of the penis and to open the channel of the shaft so that the pleasurable energy from the cock can run up into the rest of his body. From a reflexology perspective, this deep tissue awakening also stimulates and awakens all of the energy points of the rest of the body.

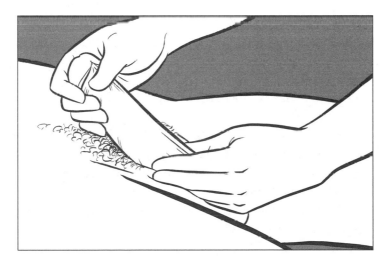

Pulling Back the Skin

Pulling Back the Skin. Here's a basic technique you'll use in many of the strokes. You'll be pulling back all the skin covering the penis, not just the foreskin. Grasp the head (glans) between thumb and fingers. Firmly stretch the cock upward until there is some resistance. (As my Chester says, "Penises are not made of china. They do not break. You are not pulling it off. You are just finding out how far it stretches.") Use your other hand to pull the loose skin down and hold it at the base where the penis meets the body. Anytime the instructions that follow tell you to "pull back the skin" or "pull back the skin and hold it at the base," this is the technique you'll use. It can be done with both circumcised and uncircumcised men. You may want to check with uncut men to find out if they want their foreskin retracted; most do.

Now it's time to sensuously apply oil or lube to the insides and tops of the thighs, making sure the cock and the balls are sufficiently oiled. Use extra lube or oil wherever there is more hair.

Rock around the Cock Clock. Lay the penis on the belly and—with both hands—stroke it from base to glans in a continuous motion. Your hands can be flat or wrapped around the shaft. Slowly move the cock from the twelve o'clock position (pointing straight up to the navel) to the one o'clock position, and so on, around the clock. At four o'clock, slide off the cock and onto the inside of the thigh, pushing energy into the leg. At six o'clock, wrap your hands around the cock. (If he is already rigidly erect, six o'clock may point straight up to the ceiling rather than downward toward the feet.) Go all the way around the clock. For some variations, go counterclockwise, or stroke your hands in opposite directions on the cock. Your left hand pulls the skin back and holds it at the base of the cock; your right hand glides out from the base, along the shaft, and grasps the glans. While the right hand hold the glans, your left hand grasps the shaft just behind the glans and glides from the back of the glans back to the base. Repeat. Continuous, slow motion makes this particularly delectable.

Twist and Shout. This is another very popular stroke. Pull back the skin with one hand, squeeze the shaft with your whole other hand, and pull with a twisting motion. As you pull, your hand will slide up the shaft and off the head. It feels best when done deeply and slowly. This stroke usually produces cringing and gasps of horror when demonstrated in front of people without penises. But really, the penis will not break. People with penises enjoy this stroke when it's done with some real intensity. Ask him. He will probably encourage you to do it harder and deeper.

The Corkscrew. This is a variation on twist and shout. You are going to pretend that the head of the cock is a cork you're trying to pop out of a wine bottle. Pull back the skin and hold it at the base. With the penis between the knuckles of your index and middle finger, squeeze, twist, and pull. You can also play with the "cork" at the end of the stroke instead of popping it off.

Fire. This is a high-energy stroke. Hold the cock straight out from his body between the flat palms of both your hands. Using lots of lube, move your hands in opposite directions with deep friction. Use medium-to-deep pressure. This can be done rapidly, or very deeply and slowly. Alternating between the two tempos usually produces loud moans of delight.

Hand Jive. This stroke is a cousin to the fire stroke. Hold the cock between both palms and interlace all your fingers. With your hands clamped together, stroke up and down the shaft. Use your thumbs to play with the head a bit. As a variation, you can hold your hands still and let him fuck your fists.

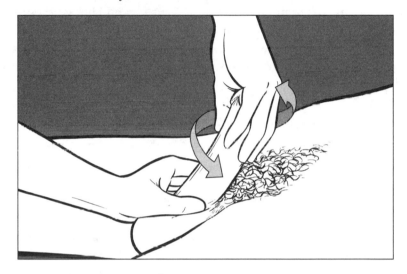

Juicer

Juicer. This is another "pull back the skin" stroke. Pull back the skin and hold it at the base. With the other hand, act as if you were juicing an orange on his cock. Use your fingertips to make a fast circular motion to "juice" up and down all along the shaft. This stroke builds and moves energy all along the shaft. When your fingers are far down on the shaft, the palm will be making slippery contact with the glans and urethral meatus (piss slit). Pay special attention to the coronal ridge (back edge of the head). You can lightly tease it with your fingernails or simply slide your fingertips all around it.

ARE WE BREATHING?

You may be giving a great massage, but are you breathing consciously? Breathe more, and it'll feel even better—to both of you. Take a long, full, deep, audible breath. This will encourage your partner to breathe. If that doesn't do it, just threaten to stop the massage until he does breathe. This is nearly 100 percent effective as a breath-maximization tool.

THIS IS NOT A HAND JOB

These cock strokes are not designed to get him off as fast as possible—quite the opposite! You want to build up a maximum amount of energy while avoiding ejaculation. To do this, use many different tempos and pressures, and change them frequently. Alternate high-energy strokes with calmer ones. Alternate strokes that focus on the glans with strokes that focus more on the shaft. Mix it up—keep him guessing! In addition, remember the body strokes. Spread that sexual energy up from his cock, into his belly and heart, and out to his arms and legs.

If at any time the receiver feels close to ejaculation, tell him to shake his body. He cannot ejaculate while he is vibrating his legs, arms, and face.

BACK TO THE COCK STROKES

Now, let's pick up where you left off. Here are some more cock strokes.

Hairy Palm. Grasp the cock with one whole hand. Grasp the base if he is erect, or hold it just behind the head if he is not. Holding the palm of your other hand flat, glide it in a light, circular motion directly on the urethral meatus. It is too intense for some men even if done lightly; other men like it quite hard. You can vary the stroke by rotating your wrist so that your flat palm glides around the meatus on the soft tissue of the glans. My favorite variation on this stroke is to hold the palm still and scrape the palm with the glans.

Heeling. This is done with the heel of your palm. Lay his cock on his belly. Place your hand flat on the penis, fingers pointed toward his feet. Using the heel of your palm, glide from the head to the base, pressing the cock into the belly. Think of the belly as an ironing board and the heel of the palm as an iron, and iron all the wrinkles out of the cock. You'll notice that when you focus the pressure on the heel of your palm, his piss slit will bend up and kiss your wrist.

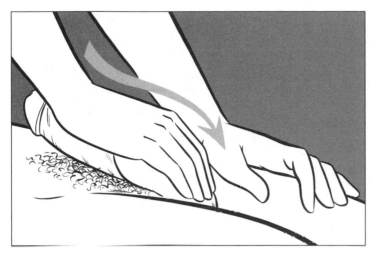

Heeling

Variations on Heeling. (1) Splay your fingers to stimulate the belly even more. (2) As your fingers approach his balls, gently wrap your fingers around them. Don't press—just give them a little light stimulation. (3) Do heeling in the opposite direction, from the base of the cock to the tip.

Cock Root Vibrations. When the cock is hard, you can feel that the erection extends all the way back up and inside the body. The perineum actually feels hard. We call this the cock root. With the fingers of one hand, lift the balls out of the way. Place the palm of your other hand against the cock root and vibrate. If he is relaxed and breathing consciously, cock root vibrations will travel up his whole body. Cock root vibrations are no different from vibrations anywhere else on the body: adjust the speed of your vibrations until you feel a natural wave.

Frenulum Frolic. The area on the underside of the head of the cock where it joins the shaft is called the frenum or frenulum. This is a very sensitive area of the penis for most men, and it is very important in the awakening and energizing process of the massage. Pinching the skin here can be very enjoyable for the receiver. You can also do thumb circles, laying the head of the penis on your palm for support, and using the tip of the thumb on your other hand to make alternating deep and very light circles on the frenum. Or both thumbs can slide over it alternately while the shaft is supported by the fingertips.

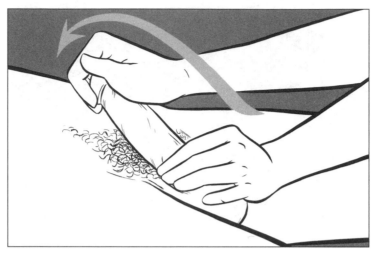

Rainbow Rub

The Rainbow Rub. This stroke also concentrates on the frenum. Pull back the skin and hold it at the base. With the other hand, grasp the glans between the fingertips and the heel of the palm. Squeeze the fingertips tightly until the hand slips up over the top of the cock. Move as though you are lifting the glans off the shaft; then put it back. This is a firm and deep stroke. The frenum (which Joseph Kramer calls the Gates of Consciousness) is thought by penis reflexologists to be the main point for stimulation of the third eye or visual center. Hence the name "rainbow rub," since it can enhance or stimulate the seeing of colors and/or visions.

REMEMBER VARIETY

Vary your strokes. The Resilient Edge of Resistance applies here as well. Just as his body gets used to a deep sensation, get light and tickle it again. When you consistently and consciously change the nature of the stimulation, the body becomes increasingly more alive and awake. Since the intention is not to ejaculate, avoid the consistent back-and-forth motion that would lead to it. But orgasms without ejaculation are permitted, and even encouraged. Constant change wakes up the penis so that it can actually become more sensitive than it would be at ejaculation. If you then move all that energy throughout the body, he can experience multiple orgasms during the course of this massage without the inevitable drain of energy that follows ejaculation.

By the way, how's the breathing going?

At this point in the massage, breathing should be full and deep and powerful. Remember, the more you breathe, the more you feel. Go for it.

Ring the Balls. This stroke is unique in its ability to delight the receiver, while cooling down the energy when ejaculation is dangerously close. Using your thumb and forefinger, form a ring around the base of the scrotal sac, where the scrotal sac joins the body. Pull the skin of the scrotal sac taut and hold it. Using the backs of your fingernails, tickle the skin. Just about the time he gets used to this tingly, tickly sensation, wrap your whole palm over the balls. When you feel him relax, go back to fingernail tickling. You can use this stroke anytime, but it is particularly effective if he is getting close to ejaculation. You can, of course, simply remove your hands from his cock—that will certainly work. But if you want to keep the energy high, "ring the balls" will keep the energy building without moving him closer to ejaculation. Stimulating the testicles sends energy streaming out through the rest of the body, so this is also an energy distribution stroke.

By now, his energy should be rockin' and rollin'. In these few minutes before the Clench and Hold, encourage him to breathe even more fully. Alternate cock strokes with body strokes. Spread the energy around his entire body. Remember, there is no goal. You are using breath and erotic energy to charge the body. Let whatever happens happen. Simply focus on building and circulating as much sexual energy as possible.

And let's get real, here. Despite your best intentions, ejaculation may happen. If it does, enjoy it! Just because it wasn't your intention doesn't make it a "mistake." It's no big deal. After all, this is erotic massage, not brain surgery. There's enough guilt around sex without piling more on ourselves. Enjoy the orgasm, and unless the receiver still wants to do a Clench and Hold, move on to the afterglow section of the massage. Later, you can make note of how you passed that point of no return and decide which techniques you'll use to avoid ejaculation the next time.

The Clench and Hold

When he is fully charged with breath and sexual energy, it's time for the Clench and Hold. Invite him to do about thirty seconds of faster, fuller breaths, followed by three big, deep breaths. He holds the third deep breath and tenses every muscle in his body, especially his buttocks and abdomen. Remember, there are a number of ways to do this clench.

He can:

* Press downward onto the massage table or floor with his hands and shoulders, head and butt, and legs and feet
* Extend his body outward as far as it can go, reaching for the opposite walls with his feet and hands
* Pull in toward the center of his body as hard as he can, first clenching his abdominal muscles, and then pulling the rest of his body in toward his abs

When he takes the third deep breath, remove your hands. Count silently to fifteen, then tell him to let go and relax.

Afterglow

Stay nearby and stay present. Even though you are not touching him, your presence is supportive. You are holding a safe space for him. Stand by the table quietly. He may be crying, laughing, or just lying very still. Unless he specifically indicates with his hands or his voice that he wants to be touched, do not touch him. Occasionally, people become very active after the Clench and Hold. If he is thrashing around on the table and you're worried about him falling off, simply place your body against the near edge of the table and reach over and grab the far edge of the table. This way, if he rolls, he won't fall off the table.

After fifteen to thirty minutes, he will probably have come back into his body. If you want to touch him, touch his knee and his wrist. This is a safe and noninvasive invitation to return to his body. Take long, slow, deep breaths, or match your breathing to his. You may want to massage him gently and slowly with a towel to remove some of the massage oil. When he indicates that he is ready to move, help him roll onto his side and, eventually, to sit up. Keep your gloves on until you are completely finished. Stay with him until you know that he is able to walk on his own two feet.

Feel free to fold, spindle, and mutilate these techniques. I recommend that you try the Erotic Awakening Massage in its entirety at least a few times in order to experience the completely unique way that breath, touch, and movement build sexual energy in this process. After that, feel free to break it apart and incorporate chunks or bits of it into other sexual play. Or, introduce other types of sexual play into the Erotic Awakening Massage. The creative possibilities are vast and the effects are extraordinary.

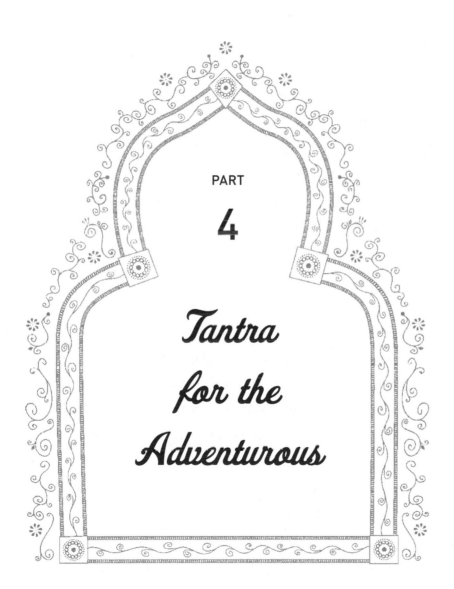

PART

4

Tantra

for the

Adventurous

Tantra continually provides new answers to the question "Is there more?" No matter where you start or where your personal path leads, your Tantric practice will inevitably present you with astonishing new sexual and spiritual adventures. As your practice deepens, you'll see new possibilities for ecstasy, both in sexual practices you have never tried and in some you may have rejected as unappealing earlier in your life. The more you live the mantra "Make no judgments, make no comparisons, and delete your need to understand," the more old prejudices will begin to drop away. Your desires will multiply and your preferences may change. Because you have changed your thinking about how sex works, you'll begin to be drawn to people and activities based more upon how conscious the person or activity is, rather than how erotic things appear at first glance.

This section of the book is designed to help you imagine and negotiate your way through some advanced erotic scenarios that can bring you great delight. In chapter 19, "Tantric BDSM," we'll look at ways to incorporate aspects of this harder-edged sacred sexuality into a Tantric practice, as well as how Tantra can expand and deepen the practice of BDSM. In chapter 20, "How to Create the Tantric Ritual That's Perfect for You," you'll learn how to create healing, satisfying, transcendent sexual moments in the midst of the challenges and occasional chaos of everyday life. In chapter 21, "Group Tantra," I'll share why some of the most satisfying sexual/spiritual experiences of my life have been in groups, and how you can try more-than-two sexual adventures without rupturing your relationship or wounding your spirit.

Think of this section as an introduction to your totality of possibilities. It's up to you when, how—and if—the possibilities become erotic reality.

CHAPTER 19

Tantric BDSM

As I mentioned in the introduction, both Tantra and BDSM are erotic arts of consciousness that have more in common than may at first seem apparent. In this chapter, I would like to encourage further blurring of the lines between Tantra and BDSM. Both BDSM and Tantra produce intense erotic sensations that can create prolonged ecstatic states of arousal and altered states of consciousness. You may have already begun to appreciate this if you have tried any of the numerous techniques and toys borrowed from BDSM that I have suggested thus far, such as bondage, sensory deprivation, and the "wilder" list of sensation producing devices (see the "Props: Mild to Wild" chart in chapter 11).

This chapter is not only for people who are new to BDSM, or who are unsure about BDSM, or who simply want to include some more intense sensation in their Tantric practice. It is also for people who love and adore BDSM and would like to know how to incorporate Tantric techniques into their play. First, however, I'd like to tell you how I stumbled upon my realization of the inseparable, yin/yang connection between these two sacred arts.

The Needle Mudra

I've always been fascinated with the idea of play piercings. Play piercings are temporary piercings. The needles are usually standard hypodermic needles, minus the syringe. These are pierced through small folds of skin anywhere on the body where there is no danger to any blood vessels, nerves, or tendons. They are designed to stay in the skin for a few minutes or a few hours. Sometimes, small weights are attached to the piercings; when the piercee moves or dances, the swinging weights stimulate the needles and the body produces endorphins. The high is euphoric.

In the Olympics of pain, I am more of a sprinter than a long-distance runner. I love the rush of endorphins from a permanent piercing: the feeling of fire when the big needle goes into my flesh, and the wait while the needle is left in place until the endorphins kick in. And then the best part: surfing the waves of altered consciousness in the afterglow. The long, meditative astral travels that accompany permanent piercings are better than any drug I have ever tried.

But I had never tried play piercings. To satisfy my curiosity, I attended a play piercing demonstration by my friend Raelyn Gallina, the high priestess of piercers. Voyeuring was the whole point of the event, held on the ninth floor of an undistinguished building in New York's Chelsea district, accessible only by a cramped, battered elevator. On the makeshift stage of what appeared to be an abandoned off-off-Broadway theatre sat two women and Raelyn. One woman was very young, probably just eighteen, with short, dark hair. She wore dark blue jeans and a dark teal zip-up sweatshirt over a neat white T-shirt. The other was older, blonde, and casually elegant in black leather pants and a satin blouse. Both were perched precariously on the edge of excitement and fear.

Raelyn is calm, centered, and entirely focused on her setup: gloves, alcohol, and needles in sealed blue packets. Every imaginable safe and hygienic protocol is in place. She is ready to begin.

The younger woman removes her sweatshirt, her T-shirt, and finally her bra. Raelyn swabs her chest with gauze soaked with alcohol. She speaks to the young woman too softly for me to hear the words. The young woman nods. Raelyn picks up the first needle. She pinches a small bit of skin on the top of the young woman's breast near the center of her chest, and pushes the needle through the flesh. The young woman winces slightly, then exhales. Raelyn waits. The young woman smiles. Two dozen needles are to follow.

One after another, Raelyn places her needles in a circular pattern, starting at the breastbone. She circles down around the outer edge of the young woman's breast, beneath her breasts, around the outer edge of the other breast, and back to the first needle at the breastbone. After each needle, Raelyn waits for the young woman to take a breath, letting the endorphins catch up with the piercings. After the first few needles, though, there's no need to wait. The young woman is clearly enjoying the effect of each subsequent needle more and more. After the last needle, Raelyn picks up a spool of elastic thread. To my amazement, she weaves the thread among the needles until the young woman is wearing a beautiful white spider web of needles and thread on her chest.

Raelyn picks up a thread in the center of the mandala and gives it a tug. I gasp. The young woman seems startled, and then a moment later she grins. The grin turns into a giddy giggle. Then she laughs. Happily.

Now it's the second woman's turn. Raelyn does exactly the same thing to her. This woman has clearly done this before. She seems less surprised by the sensations and she knows how to use her breath to increase the effect of the endorphins. It's not that she doesn't feel the pain; she appears quite sensitive. It's just that she's learned that she can play the pain like music, changing the pitch and the tone and the volume. I enjoy watching her; I know what she's doing. I use my breath the same way to build and move sexual energy in my body. I realize I'm breathing in rhythm with her. I'm getting high.

Raelyn keeps on piercing—as focused and present and beautiful as ever. Occasionally, she pauses between needles to give a gentle tug on the first woman's mandala to keep the endorphins flowing. Raelyn finishes the circle of needles on the second woman's chest, and then she weaves an identical elastic thread mandala. She gives the center threads a tug. The blonde woman shivers and then smiles.

Raelyn is sitting on a chair in the center of the stage. The first woman sits facing her on her left. The blonde woman is on her right. Raelyn playfully tugs one mandala, and then the other. Then she stands up, moves her chair away, and asks the women to move in closer to each other until their knees are almost touching. She picks up her spool of elastic thread, and my excitement grows as she ties the two webs together.

The two women are now facing each other, their chests not more than eighteen inches apart. They're gazing into each other's eyes. As if moved by some instinctual drive, they gently begin to rock back and forth, first toward one, then the other. As they become more confident, their gaze grows stronger, and their breathing becomes deeper and faster. They make an *ahh* sound on each exhale. The rocking becomes more and more active, until I see an endless wave of energy between them. I'm knocked breathless. I'm seeing something totally familiar and something completely alien at the same time. I know this! I have never had a needle mandala on my chest, but I know exactly what they're feeling. This is the Tantric heart position!

Instead of each partner touching the other's heart with the palm of their hand, these two are connected by needles and thread! Everything else is the same: the breathing, the rocking back and forth, the eye gazing. This posture can bring up laughter or tears—both of which are happening on the stage this very moment! The young dark-haired woman is smiling through the tears flowing down her cheeks and the blonde woman is simply radiant with joy.

Raelyn had woven a physical diagram of the energy exchange. Tonight, S/M had become visible Tantra! What a mindfuck! I wanted to run out and call every Tantrika I knew and tell them of my most amazing discovery. Both Tantra and this kind of S/M employ the same magic ingredients of sexual energy, endorphins, ritual, and consciousness to attain transcendent states of ecstatic connection. This was Tantra concretized. Tantra for the concrete. Urban Tantra! My head and my cunt exploded with the possibilities.

Suddenly S/M made sense to me in a way it never had before. I certainly understood that S/M ran on sexual energy and endorphins. But until tonight, I had never understood that it could be a sacred practice. But why not? The guiding principle of Tantra is "Do everything you want to do so long as you do not knowingly harm another or interfere with their spiritual growth." The guiding principle of BDSM (bondage/discipline, dominance/submission, sadism/masochism) is "Do everything you want to do so long as it's safe, sane, and consensual." The defining core of both practices is consciousness and the awareness that you are setting up a powerful dynamic for erotic or spiritual purposes. When we see both Tantra and BDSM as sacred sex, we step into the totality of possibilities of sensation and eroticism.

Five Myths about BDSM

Like Tantra, BDSM is a vastly complex and comprehensive practice incorporating a wide variety of play, from the wild to the mild. There are people who have been practicing BDSM their whole adult lives and have never played with needles or any other sharp, shiny instruments. Stories about the wilder and harder activities in BDSM can discourage people from trying any aspect, just as stories about the touchy-feely aspects of Tantra can put off people who love BDSM. Just as we have to change our minds about how sex works to understand Tantra, let's take a moment to bust some popular myths about BDSM.

MYTH #1: BDSM IS VIOLENCE. It's not hard to see how this myth began. BDSM scenes may appear scary and painful if you have never experienced this kind of play. It may seem that the dominant (a.k.a. the top, or sadist) can do anything they want to the submissive (a.k.a. the bottom, or masochist). In reality, both partners negotiate the scene before the action starts. The submissive can stop the scene at any time by uttering a "safe word."

BDSM has nothing to do with committing violence against a helpless person. Tying someone up and beating them against their will is naked brutality. It's not BDSM. BDSM operates under the all-important credo: safe, sane, and consensual. *Safe* means that precautions are taken to keep everyone involved safe from physical harm. *Sane* means that the players are not under the influence of drugs or alcohol and are not doing anything mean or malicious, and that everyone's emotional and mental safety is being cared for. *Consensual* means that everyone participating is doing so because they want to; no coercion of any kind is taking place. This means that neither partner will do lasting physical or emotional harm to the other; and neither partner will do anything to the other without their consent.

BDSM is consensual; violence is not.

MYTH #2: BDSM IS SICK. In other words, only seriously disturbed people would want to beat someone up or get beaten up.

BDSM covers a range of activities, from light bondage and role playing to sensory games and body modification. The pain level can range from intense to nonexistent. It's all up to the individuals negotiating the scene. One submissive said that the most exciting bondage her master ever put her in required no ropes, chains, or restraints of any kind. He simply had her kneel and then said two words: "Don't move."

BDSM is not an aberration. As much as 50 percent of the population is thought to have some interest in the subject, and mainstream media is full of BDSM-inspired art and erotica. Although historically BDSM behavior was listed as a psychological problem along with masturbation and homosexuality, like the latter two, it no longer is. BDSM-like practices have been performed in many cultures and by many spiritual seekers, including early Christian mystics, Native Americans, and Indian Fakirs. The energy built in these rituals can be used for spiritual journeys, as an offering to a deity, and for personal bliss.

MYTH #3: YOU COULD BE SERIOUSLY INJURED OR KILLED. True, but the same could be said of driving an automobile or walking past a construction site. BDSM is not particularly dangerous; most BDSM activities are completely safe, but some activities require more skill and practice than others. It doesn't take a federal safety inspector to figure out that playing with ropes, chains, whips, canes, electricity, and needles can be dangerous if you don't know what you're doing. This is where the safe and sane rule comes into play. If you want to play with a toy or technique you haven't used before, ask a more experienced player to teach you how to do it safely. BDSM players are extremely concerned with safety and usually are very open about sharing their expertise. If you want someone to use a particular toy on you, make sure they know how to play with it safely before you start a scene.

MYTH #4: PEOPLE WHO DO BDSM WERE ALL ABUSED AS CHILDREN. People with an interest in BDSM come from all sorts of family backgrounds, all walks of life, and all genders and sexual orientations. Some people who come from abusive backgrounds find BDSM completely unappealing; others find it to be an important part of their healing. Most BDSM aficionados come from healthy families, as do most other erotic explorers. Some identify as "lifers," having had BDSM fantasies from their earliest memories. Some players felt a connection the first time they tried BDSM and then proceeded to become regular or not-so-regular players.

MYTH # 5: BDSM HURTS TOO MUCH. Lots of people who love BDSM hate pain. Pain is not a mandatory part of any scene. Sadism/masochism involves pain, but bondage/discipline and dominance/submission can be completely pain free. Submissives who do like pain experience it in a wide variety of ways. Some receive the sting of a crop or the bite of a flogger as a kind of sexual pleasure. Some people who suffer from chronic pain claim that the focused pain they experience in S/M alleviates their chronic pain. Other people like the feeling of power they experience from being able to transmute painful stimuli into pleasure.

Consensual pain, when administered carefully, in measured doses, releases powerful endorphins that give some people a great deal of pleasure and peace.

As your practice of Tantra deepens, it is increasingly likely that you may want to expand your sexual/spiritual repertoire to include something found more commonly in a dungeon than an ashram. Go for it! It is not necessary to make a lifetime commitment to anything other than listening to your body and your spirit, and asking for what you really want and need. If on Tuesday what you want is a massage with feathers, great. If on Friday you're begging to be flogged, also great. So long as your partners agree that they are comfortable giving you what you want, go for it.

Using Tantra to Enhance BDSM

Many of the ways elements of BDSM can enhance a Tantric practice are scattered throughout this book. Here we will focus on the ways Tantra can enhance BDSM.

In 2003, I was invited by author and sex educator Tristan Taormino to facilitate two Urban Tantra workshops at Dark Odyssey, a pioneering gathering of people from the Tantric, BDSM, Polyamorous, Pagan, and Queer communities. When I stepped into the workshop room—a dungeon—for the first time, I was scared. At least half the attendees were experienced BDSM players. Although my form of Tantra welcomed a harder touch and a darker look than some Tantric practices, did it really have anything to offer people who were as devoted to BDSM as these folks?

I began by reading the quote from Osho on the subject of the three basic elements of higher sex that I shared with you in chapter 1. When I finished, both Tantrikas and BDSM players were eagerly nodding agreement. Then I noticed that everyone was nodding. I had momentarily forgotten Tantra's guiding principle: the elimination of duality. Paradoxically, the very principles that make the apparently opposing sexualities of Tantra and BDSM seem so different are the things that make them so similar.

As the weekend progressed, it became increasingly more fascinating and fun to see all the ways in which Tantra can enhance the practice of BDSM, and vice versa. Here are some actual questions I've been asked by Urban Tantra workshop participants, followed by the answers for each:

I get stage fright before I walk into a dungeon. I think about how much it is going to hurt. I love it once I start. But because of this fear, I don't play as often as I'd like. Can Tantra help me?

You are someone who needs to prepare more than usual before playing. Bottoms often wait for a top to take the lead in a scene. Your scene starts before you leave for the dungeon. Think of your BDSM scene as a Tantric ritual. Take responsibility for your own preparation. Before you leave home, chill out by doing the Bottom Breath (see chapter 4). This will help calm your fear. Then warm up: raise some endorphins and a feeling of personal power by doing a few karate chops. Or scream underwater. Or better still, do the Cathartic Meditation (see chapter 4).

Come together with your top in negotiation. In addition to talking about what you definitely would like, what you definitely don't want, and what you might be willing to try, negotiate a longer warming-up period for the rock and roll stage of your scene. Agree on a safe word. In your negotiations, also agree on how your top will treat you during the afterglow. You might want something like the kind of care provided by the giver in the Erotic Awakening Massage rituals (see chapters 16 through 18). A note for your top: a grounding hug is an excellent way to bring your bottom back to earth without losing the state of altered consciousness the two of you have spent so long building.

I'm a top. I'd like to be able to read my bottom more easily—to be more intuitive. Any tips?

Learn how to play at the Resilient Edge of Resistance (see chapter 5). No matter what kind of physical or emotional scene you are doing, you can coax more and more out of your bottom if you stay at your bottom's Resilient Edge of Resistance.

In order to stay at this ever-shifting edge, stay conscious. This simply means being in a relaxed state of awareness, with a quiet mind. Then you are able to focus gently and easily on what's going on in each present moment.

Use your breath to keep your attention focused on your intentions. Match your breath to the frequency and depth of your bottom's breath. This will bring you to a physical awareness of what they are feeling. Observe how and where their energy is moving. Are they undulating their hips and making low, guttural sounds? Then their energy is in the first or second chakras. Are they tossing their head and making high-pitched squeals? Then their energy is in the upper chakras. We build energy in BDSM in the same ways we build energy in Tantra. It's a dance of heart/upper chakra energy with genital/lower chakra energy. Keep both fires stoked with the appropriate mix of hard and soft play. Your bottom will think you can read his or her mind.

There is a top in my community that I'd love to play with. Everyone I know recommends him highly. But I just can't bring myself to play with someone I don't know well. Can Tantra help me to be more trusting?

Yes it can. In the come together/negotiation part of your ritual, do more than talk. Connect on body and spirit levels by eye gazing and using the Circular Breath. Negotiate while sitting in the Pose of Recognition with hand balancing. Play the mad/sad/glad/scared game to increase intimacy between you (see chapter 13). A few minutes of the heart position will also get your energy moving in a circuit between you. Pass this information along to your dream top . . . respectfully. If this top is as good as you hear he is, he'll love learning some new techniques.

One of my bottoms loves to jump in at the deep end with heavy sensation play right from the start. But another just can't handle that. I need some innovative tips on how to warm up my more fragile bottom.

First determine what kind of sensations the bottom likes. Thuddy? Tingly? Stinging? Sharp? Are you trying to deliver lighter strokes with the heaviest piece of equipment you have? Your fragile bottom may see that imposing tool and experience any sensation coming from it as too painful (see the "Props: Mild to Wild" chart in chapter 11). Start with an inoffensive, silly prop that delivers a milder sensation, and work your way up to harder strokes with heavier equipment. Stay at the Resilient Edge of Resistance. Drop your judgments about what is or isn't a "proper" BDSM prop. It won't spoil your tough top image if you carry a long, pink ostrich feather into the dungeon.

I can't stay in bondage very long without getting claustrophobic. I always ask to be released sooner than I want to be and sooner than my top would like. Any advice?

Try using the Bottom Breath and keep your focus on your breathing (see chapter 4). Don't use an energizing breath, and don't allow your fear to dictate the way you breathe. Short, rapid inhalations and exhalations will only make you more anxious.

Keep some part of your body moving. Even if most of your body is immobilized, there is always something you can move—your PC muscle, for example. Follow the example of my dance teacher Luigi after he was paralyzed in a car accident (see chapter 7).

I have a serious foot fetish. I fear that no one in either the Tantric or BDSM community will take me seriously. Where do I fit in?

Every fetish—from toes to tampons and plushies to playpens—can be enjoyed Tantrically. In Tantra, we strive to become the taste, feel, sound, and smell of our sensual experiences. If you love feet, dive deeply into their worship. Go into it totally. Find partners with tired toes in either the Tantric or BDSM community who will appreciate your devotion. Don't worry about fitting in. Drop your expectations of how you will be received. Don't judge yourself or allow others to judge you. Above all, drop your desire to understand why feet affect you the way they do. Conduct your foot worship with respect and consciousness and good manners, and you will be welcomed in more places than you can imagine.

I have been exclusively a top for ten years. I'm feeling out of balance. How might I use Tantra to explore bottom space?

Find yourself a switch (a partner who is comfortable either as a top or a bottom) and negotiate a scene that will be the BDSM equivalent of the Pose of Giving and Receiving position (see chapter 13). Go totally into topping and then totally into bottoming. Notice what bottoming is like for you and share that with your partner. Repeat the exercise, noticing the sense of commitment you have when you are topping. Try to move toward that sense of commitment to bottoming. Good bottoms pay attention to what their tops want from them. Using your experience as a top, pay attention to your own body responses to bottoming. Use the witnessing technique (see chapter 4).

My lover and I don't include genital sex in our BDSM play. Can I use Tantric techniques to give myself an orgasm during a scene?

Tantra and BDSM share the opportunity for extended full-body orgasmic states. In both Tantra and BDSM, these orgasmic states are created using a wide variety of techniques that go beyond genital stimulation. Practicing the Firebreath Orgasm and the Clench and Hold will open neural pathways in your body that, once opened, stay open. These newly opened energy pathways will allow more and more pleasurable sensations of all kinds to flow throughout your body. Once you can easily do the Firebreath Orgasm and the Clench and Hold, you can incorporate them into whatever kind of scene you like. While you are being flogged, for example, you can have a full-body energy orgasm by breathing sexual energy up your chakras, followed by a Clench and Hold.

I am a serious S/M player. I have a crush on someone who is far more Tantric than kinky. Is this worth pursuing? What can we do together that we would both enjoy?

Sure, it's worth pursuing, provided both of you are willing to be creative.

The Erotic Awakening Massage offers many opportunities to give and receive pleasure of varying style and intensity. Modify it to include your individual preferences.

In the next chapter, you'll find an Erotic Playsheet and directions on how to use it. It will help you to create an erotic encounter that will give each of you pleasure without asking either of you to compromise too radically.

As you can see, the yin and yang of Tantra and BDSM can be a delicious dance of conscious touch and intimate relating. Be creative. Borrow your favorite elements of each. Avoid the inclination to label your creation as a modified version of either. It's all sacred sex, and the style, intensity, and components of your creating will probably change daily. In the next chapter, you'll see how you can create rituals that will match your moods and fulfill your desires.

CHAPTER 20

How to Create the Tantric Ritual That's Perfect for You

With so many Tantric techniques available to you, how do you decide which techniques to use, and when? In this chapter, you'll learn to design Tantric rituals that fit your particular lifestyle and erotic tastes—rituals you can actually do in the time you've got. After all, life does have that sometimes pleasing, sometimes annoying tendency to present us with one surprise after another. Some are juicy and delightful; others are painful and difficult. No matter what kind of surprise happens to find you, you can use sex to celebrate it or help heal it. You accomplish this by creating erotic time that suits the mood you actually are in, as opposed to the mood you think you *should* be in order to enjoy sex.

A solo ritual is relatively simple to create, as you need only be concerned with pleasing yourself. If you have a partner and want to be sexual with them, things can get more complex. The two of you might try to come together after a busy day in the big city only to find yourselves in entirely different moods. This could lead to sex that is a compromise in which no one gets their needs met. That kind of sex can be worse than no sex at all; so over time, many couples find their sex lives fading away. Tantric rituals help you bring life, joy, and a much-needed sense of humor back to your sex life.

Whether you are planning to enjoy a Tantric ritual with your partner or by yourself, your first step is to figure out how you are feeling. This may not be as easy as it sounds. Try it. Ask yourself, "How am I feeling right at this moment?" Are you in touch with your feelings, or are you more or less clueless? Now ask yourself, "What would I enjoy sexually right now?" On my good days, I have a pretty clear idea of what would make me all wet and tingly. I can also pinpoint exactly how mad, sad, glad, or scared I am. On my stress-filled, less-than-great days, those questions make me hopelessly frustrated, and I am likely to growl, "I don't know. I'm having a hard day. I'll get back to you!"

The Erotic Playsheet

I've put together an Erotic Playsheet. It helps me get back in touch with my feelings and desires on less-than-clear days. It's a set of questions that you—or you and your partner—can answer prior to sex to get a better idea of how you are feeling and what you might want. The Erotic Playsheet is divided into two sections: how you are feeling, and which erotic activities you might enjoy. Make it part of your preparation. Breathe. Relax and take your time. The Erotic Playsheet is a gentle guide; it's not a test. Answer as many questions as you can, but leave it blank if you honestly don't know the answer or if you're not interested in a particular activity. The Erotic Playsheet is simply a tool for locating your feelings and desires so that you can better honor them.

The Erotic Playsheet

Describe your feelings and desires at this moment.

I am feeling: _____

The chakras I am most aware of are: _____

The feelings in those chakras are: _____

I definitely want: _____

I definitely don't want: _____

By the end of this ritual, I would like to feel: _____

My intention is: _____

Right now, I want to use the following techniques and props:

Breath: _____

Breath orgasm technique: _____

Erotic activity: _____

Cock massage strokes: _____

Position to fuck in: _____

Pussy massage strokes: _____

Ritual attire: _____

Ritual style: _____

Sensation-producing devices: _____

Sex toys: _____

Sounds: _____

Visualization: _____

Sensations I'd like to feel: _____

Let's follow one woman and two couples as they create Tantric rituals that satisfy their particular needs and desires.

One of Those Days

Carol is a single mother who works in sales for a large corporation. This morning, she had to leave a meeting with an important client to pick up her son at his school and take him to the hospital because he got into a fight and broke his wrist. This afternoon, Carol was reprimanded by her boss, who questioned her commitment to the company. She got a lecture from her son's principal about her parenting skills. And she got a call from her lover, Sonia, who wonders why Carol can't spend more time with her.

On the opposite page you can see how Carol filled out her Erotic Playsheet when she finally got home.

To chill out, Carol draws a warm bath scented with essential oil of ylang-ylang. To warm up, she takes a deep breath, puts her face in the water, and screams "Fuck you!" at her boss and at the school principal. She takes another breath, puts her face in the water, and screams "You asshole!" at her son. Her third breath and scream is at her girlfriend: "Leave me alone!" Feeling considerably less tense and numb, Carol goes to her bedroom and locks the door. She lights her favorite rose-scented candle, opens the window for some fresh air, and puts *Pearl* in the CD player.

As she gets out her vibrator and her favorite dildo, she realizes that *Pearl* is not quite the right music for the come together section of her ritual. She puts ten minutes of a sensuous Brazilian instrumental on the CD player, with *Pearl* programmed to play right afterward.

Carol lies on her bed and begins the simplified Firebreath Orgasm. As she begins breathing into her solar plexus, Carol discovers she can't even feel this part of her body. After several breaths, she begins to cry. She keeps on breathing, and the tears keep on flowing. As the energy moves up into her heart, her crying subsides and she feels the stirring of a warm, comforting fullness in her solar plexus.

As she breathes into her throat, *Pearl* begins. Janis wails "Move Over" as Carol sucks and tongues her dildo to lubricate it; then she slides it into her vagina. She turns her vibrator on high and places it on the exposed end of the dildo. As the rock and roll phase intensifies, Carol rolls over onto her hands and knees, breathing, Kegeling, vibrating her clitoris, and undulating her body like a wave. After her first orgasm, she rolls onto her back and keeps up her circular breathing. When her clitoris has become

Carol's Erotic Playsheet

Describe your feelings and desires at this moment.

I am feeling: Exhausted, drained, angry.

The chakras I am most aware of are: Solar plexus.

The feelings in those chakras are: Caved-in, hollow, empty.

I definitely want: A clitoral orgasm with G-spot stimulation.

I definitely don't want: Anyone else around.

By the end of this ritual, I would like to feel: Centered, powerful, at peace.

My intention is: To take back my power.

Right now, I want to use the following techniques and props:

Breath: Circular Breath.

Breath orgasm technique: Simplified Firebreath Orgasm.

Erotic activity: Selfloving.

Cock massage strokes: N/A.

Position to fuck in: Lying on my back. Maybe doggie style if I feel up to it.

Pussy massage strokes: None.

Ritual attire: Nothing.

Ritual style: Simple, short, and solo.

Sensation-producing devices: Electric vibrator.

Sex toys: Large dildo.

Sounds: I want to listen to Janis Joplin's Pearl CD as loudly as I can get away with.

Visualization: Janis Joplin's freedom, power, and resilience entering my solar plexus.

Sensations I'd like to feel: Intensity.

less sensitive, Carol brings herself to orgasm again, this time combining her orgasm with a Clench and Hold.

When Carol lets go after the Clench and Hold, she lies flat on her back with her palms up, in the classic yoga corpse pose. In the afterglow, Carol meditates as Janis sings about freedom being just another word for nothing left to lose. Carol realizes that she does feel free, strong, and quite peaceful. By the time Janis asks the Lord for a Mercedes Benz, Carol is dozing off with a satisfied smile on her face.

Different Lives

Tiffany and Grant have been live-in lovers for two years. For the past four years, Tiffany has been working as a dominatrix to pay her way through drama school in New York. She earns a substantial amount of money and she enjoys her work. It has helped her develop and expand her sense of personal and sexual power.

Recently, however, Tiffany has been feeling out of balance. She is trying to connect more with her compassionate, intuitive, spiritual side. Earlier this week, Tiffany auditioned for and was cast in a supporting role in an independent film to be shot in Los Angeles. Having recently graduated, Tiffany feels it's time to change careers and move to L.A. She is thrilled with her new acting job, but apprehensive about all the changes that this will bring.

Grant is a writer. He has written two books of critical essays, both of which were published and well received. His dream is to be a best-selling novelist. He has spent the better part of the past year writing an erotic thriller for which he had high hopes. This week, his agent informed him that three publishers turned down the book, calling it too cerebral, theoretical, unrealistic, and unsexy. Grant has no objections to relocating to Los Angeles to be with Tiffany. However, he is better at planning than at execution, and he has no idea how to actually go about making the move. At home one evening in new York, they decide to share a Tantric ritual. You can see Tiffany and Grant's Erotic Playsheets on the following pages.

Tiffany and Grant show each other their playsheets. They laugh at the obvious differences in their needs and desires. It only takes a few minutes of loving negotiation to arrive at a ritual that will satisfy them both. They begin by setting the stage. They light candles and gather massage supplies, glasses of water, and some fruit. Tiffany puts soft, pretty pillows on the floor and dresses herself in a colorful sarong while Grant changes into his leather shorts. They put music by Vangelis, Enigma, and Stan Getz on the CD player and set the play to random.

Tiffany's Erotic Playsheet

Describe your feelings and desires at this moment.

I am feeling: Excited, scared.

The chakras I am most aware of are: Root and sex chakras.

The feelings in those chakras are: Horny, urgent.

I definitely want: To fuck.

I definitely don't want: Any BDSM.

By the end of this ritual, I would like to feel: Softer, gentler, more open.

My intention is: To bring my sexual energy up into my heart and my third eye. To open up and activate my heart and my intuition.

Right now, I want to use the following techniques and props:

Breath: Heart Breath and Breath of Fire.

Breath orgasm technique: None.

Erotic activity: Partner sex.

Cock massage strokes: N/A.

Position to fuck in: Any.

Pussy massage strokes: G-spot strokes, rock around the clit clock, divine drumming.

Ritual attire: Silk sarong, but not for long!

Ritual style: Soft, intimate.

Sensation-producing devices: Fingers and cock.

Sex toys: None.

Sounds: Music that's big and dramatic and a bit otherworldly.

Visualization: Hot fire moving into my heart and upper chakras and cool water flowing down into my lower chakras.

Sensations I'd like to feel: Stroking, sensual.

Grant's Erotic Playsheet

Describe your feelings and desires at this moment.

I am feeling: Confused, frightened.

The chakras I am most aware of are: Throat and third eye.

The feelings in those chakras are: My throat feels tight and I have a headache.

I definitely want: To be blindfolded and restrained.

I definitely don't want: Any pain.

By the end of this ritual, I would like to feel: Stronger, grounded, more in my body.

My intention is: To feel my entire body.

Right now, I want to use the following techniques and props:

Breath: Bottom Breath and Heart Breath.

Breath orgasm technique: Clench and Hold.

Erotic activity: Partner sex.

Cock massage strokes: Fire, rainbow rub, twist and shout, rock around the cock clock.

Position to fuck in: Tiffany on top.

Pussy massage strokes: N/A.

Ritual attire: My leather shorts.

Ritual style: Don't know.

Sensation-producing devices: Mouth, hands, pussy.

Sex toys: None.

Sounds: Jazz or instrumental.

Visualization: My sexual energy is coming into my cock from a root that extends into the hot molten center of the earth.

Sensations I'd like to feel: Tiffany's mouth on my cock.

To chill out, both do ten minutes of the shaking section of the Exhilaration Meditation with their eyes closed. For their warm up, they give each other grounding hugs. To come together, they sit facing each other on the floor. After a couple of minutes of eye gazing, each shares the things they are mad, sad, glad, or scared about while the other listens silently. They follow this with the Pose of Giving and Receiving. Tiffany receives first. On some of the strokes, Grant uses a feather and a bit of fur instead of his fingers. When it is Grant's turn to receive, Tiffany blindfolds him and ties his hands in front of him. She feeds him, teasing him with each bite. She pauses, making him wonder and wait for what will come next. She softly strokes his head and neck, then rakes her fingernails down his arms and onto his thighs.

Tiffany tells Grant to lie back on the floor. Rock and roll begins as she takes off his shorts and kisses his cock. She runs her tongue around his cock and sucks it until he is hard and breathing deeply. Then she lubes her hands, places them on either side of Grant's cock, and gives him particularly hot fire strokes. She follows this with all the strokes he requested, plus a few extra, just for fun. Then she kisses him, removes his blindfold, unties his hands, and says, "My turn."

Grant rolls her over onto her back and strokes her breasts, kissing her nipples. His hands move down her belly to her pussy. He begins pussy petting. Then he begins to rock around the clit clock, throwing in an occasional pinch and pull. He does some tap, tap tapping for divine drumming, and then, since Tiffany asked for harder strokes, he plays her like a big bass drum, one big beat at a time. As her squeals of laughter and pleasure subside, he gently and slowly slips a finger inside her vagina and holds it perfectly still. Tiffany begins to move against his hand, then she asks for another finger. He complies, giving her G-spot a yummy, intense massage, just the way she likes it.

Tiffany sits up and straddles Grant in Yab Yum. They fuck blissfully and deeply in this position, breathing and Kegeling. Grant begins to breathe faster, fuller breaths that let Tiffany know he wants to do a Clench and Hold with her. They take in a deep breath, clench, stare into each other's eyes, and then let go. They gaze into each other's eyes; it is as if they can see into each other's soul. Finally, they gently fall backward into Heart-Foot-Hand position. In their afterglow, Grant feels his root chakra pressed against Tiffany's, and her power and earthiness supporting him. Tiffany feels Grant's foot on her heart and feels her heart and third eye alive, awake, and pulsing. They lie like this for many minutes. When they sit up, they wrap a blanket around themselves, sip some water, and feel closer, stronger, more open, and more trusting with each other and about their new life.

P.S., Your Cat Is Dead

Simon and Tony have been lovers for four years. This past year, Tony went through major surgery. Simon took time off from his job to nurse him back to health. Just as Tony was feeling better, Simon's mother was diagnosed with cancer and died within three months. Two weeks ago, Simon's only brother was killed in an automobile accident. Tony and Simon are trying to cope. They love each other and they believe in the power of sex to heal. Simon and Tony's Erotic Playsheets are on the next two pages.

Tony sets up their massage table in the bedroom. He turns off all the lamps and lights just enough candles to be able to see. He turns on an electric heater. When the room is comfortably warm, he puts *Thunderdrums* into the CD player and invites Simon into the room.

Seeing how stiff Simon looks, Tony invites him to chill out with an elephant massage. It makes Simon feel looser, and he even laughs a little. When Simon stands up, he offers Tony an elephant massage, and Tony accepts. Tony suggests that Simon might like to warm up by doing a section of the Cathartic Meditation, which they both enjoy. Simon doesn't feel up to it, but he wants to let out some of the anger he is feeling. So he yells as he throws karate chops into a pillow that Tony holds in front of him. Tony yells along with Simon, which lets Simon feel supported and also gets Tony's energy rising.

To come together, Tony and Simon sit facing each other on their massage table. They gaze into each other's eyes. Tony tells Simon how much he loves him, how grateful he is for all the love and support Simon has given him this past year, and that it is his intention to do the same for him now. Simon gratefully accepts and asks Tony if it will be okay if they call in the spirits of Simon's mother and brother. Tony thinks it is a wonderful idea and suggests they also invite in the spirits of some of their friends who have passed away. Simon and Tony call out the names of their loved ones and invite their spirits to join them in their ritual.

Simon lies on his belly on the massage table. Tony begins by giving him a sensual massage. Although it feels nice, Simon tells Tony that he needs something harder. Tony chooses a medium-intensity flogger and begins striking Simon's back and buttocks and thighs. Simon asks for harder strokes. Although he specifically asked for no pain, he experiences the flogging as delicious. Simon takes deeper and deeper breaths; they feel like the first deep breaths he has taken in weeks. Tony, watching Simon's breathing and body, slows down, doing fewer, more intense strokes. The last strokes take most of Tony's strength. Simon sighs deeply and moans. Finally, Tony puts down the flogger and picks up the massage oil.

Simon's Erotic Playsheet

Describe your feelings and desires at this moment.

I am feeling: Distraught, helpless, lost, hypersensitive. It feels like every nerve in my body is numb and raw.

The chakras I am most aware of are: Heart, chest.

The feelings in those chakras are: Heavy, congested.

I definitely want: To stop hurting.

I definitely don't want: More pain.

By the end of this ritual, I would like to feel: Peaceful.

My intention is: To accept Tony's love and support.

Right now, I want to use the following techniques and props:

Breath: Bottom Breath and Circular Breath.

Breath orgasm technique: Clench and Hold.

Erotic activity: Not sure, maybe erotic massage.

Cock massage strokes: Any or all are good.

Position to fuck in: Not sure if I want to fuck.

Pussy massage strokes: N/A.

Ritual attire: Something to keep warm; I'm having chills.

Ritual style: Dark, quiet, wordless.

Sensation-producing devices: Whatever works.

Sex toys: None.

Sounds: Drums.

Visualization: I want to visualize a strong, eternal connection with my mother's and my brother's spirits.

Sensations I'd like to feel: Strong, intense.

Tony's Erotic Playsheet

Describe your feelings and desires at this moment.

I am feeling: Helpless with regard to Simon's pain. Anxious.

The chakras I am most aware of are: Heart.

The feelings in those chakras are: Love, compassion, sadness.

I definitely want: To help Simon feel lighter.

I definitely don't want: To make things any worse.

By the end of this ritual, I would like to feel: Happy, helpful.

My intention is: To give comfort and support to Simon.

Right now, I want to use the following techniques and props:

Breath: I want to do the Circular Breath and the Bottom Breath.

Breath orgasm technique: N/A.

Erotic activity: I'd like to give an erotic massage to Simon.

Cock massage strokes: I'll give any/all that Simon would like.

Position to fuck in: N/A.

Pussy massage strokes: N/A.

Ritual attire: Nothing.

Ritual style: Dark, intense.

Sensation-producing devices: Whatever Simon wants. I might try a thudder and a flogger.

Sex toys: Whatever Simon wants.

Sounds: New age, ethereal.

Visualization: My love and support for Simon flowing from my cock, through my heart, and into my hands as I touch him.

Sensations I'd like to feel: Open and present in my giving.

Simon feels his nerves begin to calm down. He is ready to rock and roll. As Tony starts to oil his cock, Simon realizes how little he has been feeling, not only in his cock but everywhere in his body. Tony concentrates on intense, energy-building cock strokes. Every time Simon gets close to ejaculating, Tony removes his hands from Simon's cock and spreads the energy up into his heart. Tony visualizes all their combined sexual energy flowing into Simon's body, replacing his grief and anger with peace and joy. He feels that he is channeling the love of all the spirits they have called in. Simon tells Tony he wants to do a Clench and Hold. They breathe fast, full breaths together, and then Simon clenches, holding the clench so long that Tony has to tell him to let go.

At first Simon is very still. Then he begins to smile. Tears run down his cheeks and onto the sheet covering the massage table. Tony stands by the table, just being present. After a few minutes, Tony asks Simon if he'd like to be covered. Simon says yes.

After Tony covers Simon, he changes the music, replacing *Thunderdrums* with soft, celestial music. Simon lies perfectly still. He is so still that Tony is not even sure he is breathing. Tony just sits with him. He feels the presence of the family and friends they have invited to join them as if they are alive and standing beside them in the room. It is profoundly peaceful and comforting. Tony weeps.

Meanwhile, Simon does indeed feel as if he is dead. He isn't aware of any specific images or sounds, though he does remember thinking that he didn't know it was possible to breathe so shallowly. He starts to giggle. His giggles become peals of laughter, which in turn become wracking sobs, as he recognizes the overwhelmingly strong presence of his mother and his brother. He realizes that he has not laughed so hard since he was with the two of them last year. Simon thanks them both and tells them how much he loves and misses them. For the first time since their deaths, he feels the comfort of knowing that they will always be with him.

Tony and Simon sit in their separate but shared afterglow for almost an hour. Finally, Simon offers Tony his hand. Holding hands, they do not speak. When Simon is ready to get off the massage table, Tony takes him into the bathroom and the two of them share a warm bubble bath by candlelight. Both Tony and Simon have received a healing.

No matter what your day, week, or month has brought you, you can create a Tantric ritual that will transport you from whatever you're feeling now into someplace more ecstatic and peaceful. Make some copies of the Erotic Playsheet. Fill it out and start creating your own rituals. Be flexible. In the three examples given, the resulting rituals did not precisely follow what was written on the playsheets. The rituals morphed into what the participants wanted and needed in the present moment. Stay conscious. Honor your intentions. Remember to celebrate.

CHAPTER 21

Group Tantra

Sex in groups is vastly underrated and underexplored. The consensus in polite society has always been that sex is a private affair; only exhibitionists and sex workers are brazen enough to be sexual in public.

Wrong.

Many people harbor fantasies about having sex in public. Fantasies such as fucking in an elevator or in a dark corner of a museum turn us on because of the danger of being discovered. Public sex is such a powerfully "bad" thing to do. But there is another, more subtle, force at play. Public sex owes its power to the presence—real or imagined—of other people. Think about how sexual energy builds in your body when you are alone; then think about how it builds when you are with a partner. For most people, the presence of another being amplifies the energy, causing it to build more quickly and intensely. Adding more beings to the party can exponentially increase the intensity, the power, and the magic of an erotic encounter. Notice that I say adding partners *can* increase the intensity, not that it always will. Building erotic energy in groups is tricky. Actually, it's not building the energy that is tricky, it's building the group that takes consciousness, intention, and attention.

In 1977, a swingers' club for heterosexual couples opened in New York City. Plato's Retreat was legendary; it had a sixty-person Jacuzzi, a clothing-optional dance floor, hot and cold buffets, and a huge orgy room. Plato's Retreat was less than thirty blocks from my apartment for eight years, and yet I never went. For my taste, it was overwhelmingly heterosexual, and I wasn't particularly interested in heterosexual sex. What's more, I'd heard that the kind of sex that went on there was pretty sleazy, chaotic, and unsafe on an emotional as well a physical level. The very few swingers I had met up to that point just weren't people with whom I wanted to be sexual. Even though I was very curious about group sex, I imagined that all group sex parties would be like Plato's Retreat, so I stayed away from all of them. Years later—after I had begun to practice Tantra—I was finally able to articulate what I had been trying to avoid. More important, I had discovered what kind of group sexual energy I loved and wanted more of. I had found my erotic group preference when I started participating in, and later facilitating, sex workshops.

Why would a sex workshop be hotter than a sex party? It might seem at first glance that the casual, unstructured nature of a party would be more conducive to a hot time than a workshop. Paradoxically, the casual, drop-in nature of most sex parties or BDSM play parties can be an erotic disadvantage because their structure and style are modeled more on a party than on a ritual or a workshop. In most cases, the organizers of the party find a space for six to eight hours or so on a given evening. They send out invitations to the general public or to a large mailing list, and anyone can come to the party. This system is great for bringing new people and fresh energy to an ongoing party group, but the downside is getting a lot of people who want to play but don't know anyone else in the room. As at many regular parties, people wind up hiding in the corners, clutching their drinks, and staring at the action in the center of the room. And while it is true that sex with a stranger at a party like this can be very hot, it is not the same as participating in group erotic energy. Conscious group erotic energy has to be built over time by everyone in the room, and most play parties don't last long enough to build that kind of energy.

Let's compare this to a sex workshop. All my workshops that involve actual sexual contact between the participants have lasted at least two or, more commonly, three days. Whenever possible, we find a venue in a beautiful natural setting. The first day is primarily devoted to getting to know each other. We sit in a circle, agree to abide by some basic rules of behavior and manners, and discuss what we hope to get out of the weekend. We do some moving meditations to release any stress and negative feelings we may have brought with us from our daily lives. Everyone learns various ways to breathe and to move erotic energy around. Everyone receives some instruction on how to touch with conscious intention. Then we all get to give and receive a sensual massage. That is just day one!

When we meet again the next morning, after a good night's sleep, people are still a bit nervous about being sexual in a group but are willing to let go and try it because the other participants are no longer strangers. They are people we have all come to know and trust—at least for the duration of the workshop. For the next two days, we can practice truly conscious sex, because we share common tools, an agreed-upon safer-sex protocol, and a sense of safety. Everyone has had the time to set their own boundaries and has agreed to respect the boundaries of others.

How can we experience the goodies of a workshop in the time and space of a party? It is certainly possible to have conscious sex in a group setting that isn't three hours away and doesn't last three days. There are countless ways to be sexual in a group. Sex in groups does not have to mean having sex with everyone else in the group. Masturbation can be a group activity; so can partner sex. You can even adapt the traditional Tantric partner positions to accommodate triads, so that the third person never has to sit out and wait their turn for a partner. Be creative and inclusive!

How to Throw a Great Ritual/Sex Party

1. Articulate an intention for your ritual. "I want to get off with as many people all over me as possible" is a perfectly lovely desire, but it's a lousy intention for a group ritual. Your intention should include and benefit all members of the group. For example: "Our intention is to bring together members of the S/M and Tantric communities for an evening-long exploration of the sacred eroticism common to both." Your intention should be stated in a sentence or two. Keep it simple.

2. What kind of erotic play suits your intention? What doesn't? Be specific. Is nudity expected? Required? Optional? Is fucking allowed? How about blood sports, such as play piercings? Decide in advance what is and isn't acceptable for your group. Make sure to provide a safe, comfortable space for all the activities you plan to encourage.

3. Before the ritual, inform everyone of the rules/protocols for the ritual. Be sure to clearly state, in advance, your intention and your safer-sex policy, so that people will come mentally and physically prepared. Of course, you will have safer-sex supplies at easy-to-reach locales throughout your space.

4. Have a facilitator. Or a team of facilitators. At least one facilitator who is not participating in the fun is needed to make sure that the rules are being followed and no one is getting hurt. We call this job "holding the space." You might call your facilitator a Dungeon Master or a High Priestess. Choose a title appropriate to the style of your ritual. In one of my workshops, the person who made sure participants followed the safer-sex protocol was called "Proto-Kali."

5. Start and end at a specified time. Ask everyone to arrive before the start time; people should not be allowed to drop in once the ritual gets going. Anyone who leaves early must tell the facilitator they are leaving. Looking up from a hot time, realizing someone is missing, and not knowing why can completely break an erotic spell.

6. Gather with clothes on first. Whether it's a meal, a circle, or some other way of gathering, make sure everyone gets to meet everyone else and share their expectations for the gathering. Let people ask questions. Restate the rules and the intention. People feel safer when they see that everyone else hears and agrees to the same rules.

7. Be flexible but firm. Keep true to your intention. Remember, this is your party. If someone isn't enjoying themselves, it is perfectly okay for them to leave. Take note of things that work and things that don't so that you can make your next party/ritual even better.

Club Relate

Lynda Gayle and her husband, Tom, are the founders of Club Relate, America's first heterosexual masturbation club. The story of Club Relate is a fine example of how careful planning, effective rules, and good manners create a great time for everyone. Lynda's story is also a great lesson in how to create a sex party that respects people's relationships, feelings, and desires.

My husband, Tom, and I used to go to swingers' clubs. Both of us particularly enjoy masturbation, but at the swingers' clubs it was a real taboo. It's hard to believe that masturbation would be looked down upon in that scene, but it is just not an okay thing to do. I think it's because of the intensity of the act. And when people are not okay with masturbation in their own lives, they don't want to see anybody else doing it.

We placed a personal ad to see if there were other people who also enjoyed masturbation who would like to join us. Thirteen people showed up for the first party. It was the first time everyone had gotten together with a group of people where it was okay to do this. It was like . . . magic! We started at 4 p.m. and went until 4 o'clock in the morning! Needless to say, we were all exhausted. I told Tom, we have got to figure out a better way of doing this! So now parties have set time limits.

The time limits also help make our club relationship-protective. If you go to a swingers' party, your wife might go with someone and stay for an hour . . . two hours . . . three hours . . . that can make you a little anxious! At Club Relate, everything is done together in the open. Everything is structured so that you know when it starts and when it stops. And because everything is done together there is no secretiveness.

At first, we were meeting people individually before they came to the party. But pretty soon there were so many people that individual interviews were impractical. Now we have group orientations for the new people in the afternoon before each party starts. We spend some time talking about why masturbation is important in their lives, if they were ever made to feel guilty about it, and, perhaps most important, if they are able to share it in their primary relationship at this time. Then we go over the rules for the club and how the party works. There are two rules. The first rule is: no drugs in ya, on ya, or around ya. The second rule is: if anyone asks you if you want to play and it's not what you want, you don't have to be creative and come up with an excuse. All you have to say is, "No, thank you, but thank you for asking."

After the orientation, we go to dinner. The people who have already been through the orientation know we go to dinner at 5 p.m. So they come and have dinner with the new people. There's nothing like getting to know people over dinner. Then we come back to the hotel—the parties usually take place in a penthouse suite—at about 7:30 for hospitality time. During this time, we get people talking about where they have come from. We have had people from Italy, England, Germany, and Sweden, as well as from all over the U.S. It really is incredible how far people travel. Usually we have thirty-five to forty people at a party; we will not go over fifty. We try to keep a balanced ratio between couples, single females, and single males.

After hospitality time, everyone is told that it is time to dress down. That means you get out of your street clothes into something sexy, or if you are okay with your body and you feel sexy when you are nude, then great! Then the party starts. It lasts for one hour and fifteen minutes. I know that doesn't sound very long, but the party is relationship-protective. If somebody is with your partner, they are not going to be with them for longer than an hour and fifteen minutes. Also, we don't allow smoking at our parties and we figured people could go an hour and fifteen minutes without a smoke. In a way, it's just like kindergarten—we tell you when it's time to rest, have something to eat and drink, and freshen up.

We have a thirty-minute break and then Tom announces, "It's time to start the second session." This session also lasts for an hour and fifteen minutes. We finish at around 11:30 p.m. This way it's still early if you want to invite someone back to your room for a private session. Or if you want to drive back home.

Masturbation is not the only thing that goes on at our parties. To me, masturbation is self-stimulation or some kind of manual stimulation. It is not intercourse. If you use a dildo or a vibrator, that is masturbation, whether you are holding it or someone else is. There are some people who only want to watch . . . and some people who want to be watched. There are some couples who want to have intercourse with each other while everyone is watching—that is really hot. I love watching people watch that! I say that any kind of sex play is acceptable because there is always somebody who wants to watch it.

Sometimes we might have some light S/M (which we call Sensual Magic). There might be people who didn't know that they wanted to be spanked, but when they see it, it's a turn-on. A wife may say to her husband, "Hey, that's what I want you to do to me." So in a way, it's like a class or show-and-tell. Plus, you get to move around from room to room. Usually there are at least two bedrooms. In one particular hotel we go to, the closet is big enough for a party! Plus, the bathroom has a shower and a Jacuzzi.

I asked Lynda Gayle what advice she would give to someone who'd like to try swinging but might not know how to start—or might be a little afraid.

> I would say: do it anyway. Go armed with Rule #2: "No, thank you, but thank you for asking." Also, go with a clear idea of what you do—and do not—want to experience. State what your limits are to others so they will know how to respect them; but do tell them what it is you do want to experience. Even if you just want to watch your wife touch another woman's breast for the first time, say that! Somebody is going to help you find that experience because they want you to have fun. For the most part, the people you are going to find in the swinging lifestyle are very sincere and kind. If that's not what you find at your first club, keep looking.

Happy Birthday

Another delicious and powerful way to manifest group sexual energy is in a ritual performed by a group to pleasure one person. It can be a ritual to celebrate a birthday or to mark an important life passage, or it can be a kind of shamanic ritual to help someone find a new life path.

My friend Margaret wanted to do something special for her girlfriend Robin's thirty-fifth birthday. So, on the evening of Robin's birthday, four of us arrived at Margaret's apartment dressed in high slut gear and wearing elaborate masks. When the unsuspecting Robin arrived, she tried to hide her delight as we blindfolded her, removed her clothes, tied her hands behind her back, and covered her with an oversized coat. We took off our masks, put on coats over our slut outfits, and walked Robin outside to my car, which was waiting up the block. We worried about being stopped by some good samaritan who thought we were kidnapping her. Luckily, Margaret lived across the street from the Gay/Lesbian/Bisexual/Transgender Community Center, so the only attention we attracted was from a lovely queer man who said, "*Ooo*, is it a birthday kidnapping? How fun!"

We drove the blindfolded Robin into, out of, and around the twisted streets of Greenwich Village for something approaching an hour. She never knew until later that she had only gone across town. We threatened her with all manner of devilish things that we would do to her whether or not she behaved. When we finally arrived at the East Village loft of one of the kidnappers, we hustled her up several flights of stairs and into the bedroom. We tied her spread-eagled to the bed and turned up the music in the room as loud as we thought we could get away with without complaints from the neighbors. This gave us time to prepare for the next part of our plan while Robin, bound and blindfolded in the next room, could not possibly hear what we were doing or saying.

Margaret had carefully orchestrated the ritual to fulfill as many of Robin's desires and fantasies as possible. We began in the bedroom, stroking Robin with some soft and some not-so-soft floggers. We played her body like a percussion instrument, which she very much appreciated. Robin is a world-class drummer. We used every imaginable sensation-producing device we could find: hard, thuddy things and sharp, stingy things; soft, fuzzy things and cool, smooth things. We played her fast and hard, then soft and slow, then slow and hard. In between, we teased her with nibbles of tiny champagne grapes and chocolate.

After this act of our birthday ritual had reached its climax, we let her rest, giving her body time to integrate and appreciate all the delicious sensations with which we had bombarded her. Then we untied her and carried her into a big sunken tub. Her lover held her like a baby as we all bathed and caressed her. Slowly, we removed her blindfold. The dark marble bathroom was the showpiece of this loft. It looked like a cave temple, decorated with candles placed judiciously around the room. Robin looked as though she had been reborn.

After Robin's long, luxurious bath, we all wrapped her in a warm soft towel and brought her into the main room for a snack of delicious gourmet treats. Robin was in bliss. She thanked us all profusely, obviously thinking that her surprise was over. "Oh no," we informed her. "We were just giving you a little break before the big finale: an Erotic Awakening Massage given by all five of us!"

An Erotic Rite

I delight in designing and facilitating a group erotic ritual for someone I love. One of my lovers, Diana, had long admired my labia piercings and decided she wanted one. She wanted to receive the piercing, not at a traditional piercing parlor, but as part of a ritual in a workshop setting. The Erotic Rites workshop was perfect. In it, each woman designed a ritual or rite for herself. The intention of the rite was to receive support and assistance from the group in a ritual that would honor the woman's sexual past as it prepared her to step into her erotic future. Roughly half the group assisted each woman in her ritual; the rest witnessed the rite.

Diana and I had just begun our relationship. She had been married to a man for twenty-five years and was now, with her husband's encouragement, exploring both polyamory and sex with a woman. Needless to say, Diana was at the doorway to a hugely significant new phase of her sexual evolution.

Diana and I began her ritual seated and facing each other on a massage table in the Yab Yum position. We breathed together, gazed into each other's eyes, and shared how much we loved each other and what we wanted for each other. Diana stated her intention of what she wanted to receive from her ritual. I stated what I hoped to give her. We breathed ourselves into a seated, open-eyed Clench and Hold. I gently laid her back onto the massage table, removed her bra and panties, and kissed her over her heart chakra. When Diana told me she was ready, I called over the professional piercer, who was standing by. As the needle pierced her labia, Diana let out a low, guttural sound, then opened her eyes in amazement as the warm rush of endorphins flowed up her body. After the piercer put in the jeweled ring Diana had selected, Diana sat up and looked at it, beaming with pride and pleasure. Having raised all her yummy endorphins, we were now about to put them to good use.

As Tina Turner's "Never in Your Wildest Dreams" played in the background, six women massaged Diana, alternating elegant, sensual strokes using hands and feathers with hard, slapping strokes using wooden spoons and light floggers. They stroked her everywhere but between her legs where the fresh piercing was. As the music changed to Gloria Gaynor's "I Will Survive," we began vibrating her chakras with two huge electric vibrators. We skipped the root chakra, which was too close to the fresh piercing. We breathed with her and danced beside the table, sending her all the love and juice and energy we could. Meanwhile, the women who were witnessing the ritual surrounded us, dancing and generating more energy.

Caught in the tsunami of energy we were all creating, Diana was breathing rapidly. Suddenly she took a huge, deep breath and held it in a Clench and Hold. We screamed "Go for it! Reach right into the next part of your life!" Diana let go. Her spine arched like a bow. As it curled back down to the table, her legs arched. Then, as they came back down, she sat up and curled up over her legs. She looked like a sea serpent riding a wave. She hugged herself; she stroked herself; she cried. She appeared to pass seamlessly through veils of emotions as though she were traveling through the past, present, and future of her life. Finally she lay still and peaceful on the table. She opened her eyes and reached for me. I fell into her arms, crying.

You do not need to wait for a workshop to create an experience like this for yourself or your lover. You can gather a group of friends together and create an erotic ritual in your own home. If being sexual around friends who you do not consider lovers is unfamiliar to you, it may seem strange or uncomfortable. Our culture saturates itself with sex. At the same time, it makes rules to keep sex confined to one primary relationship. Silly, huh? Why should we not play sexually with our dearest friends? Sure, perhaps not all your friends would be interested in that kind of play, but it's not hard to make friends who would be. "Fuck buddies" are friends who get together to enjoy sex the way other friends may get together to see movies or play sports.

A Weekend in the Country

One of my favorite sex parties with friends was a celebration of the completion of a project we had all worked on together. On Earth Day in 1990, I got together with nine other graduates of Betty Dodson's Bodysex workshops to make a video documenting Betty's twenty-five years of legendary masturbation workshops for women. The result was *Selfloving: Portrait of a Women's Sexuality Seminar.* (See the resources section at the end of the book for information about how to order a copy.) The video shoot was a smashing success, and all the women who participated became good friends. A few weeks after the shoot, one of the women asked us all to a slumber party at her new home in a suburban town in New England. Six of us were available and eagerly accepted. When we asked if we could bring anything, our hostess, Julie, said, "Yes. Your vibrators, a sexy outfit, and whichever dildo you're the fondest of this week."

We arrived in the late afternoon of a warm spring Saturday. Our visit started suburbanly enough. Julie took us on a tour of her beautiful old colonial house and served us iced tea, and we all sat down to catch up with each other's news. As the afternoon turned into evening, our hostess invited us to gather around the dining room table for hors d'oeuvres and entertainment. We proceeded to suck down huge, salty, raw oysters as our hostess climbed onto the table, smiling down at us seductively. She performed an extremely athletic and explicit striptease, giving each of us a tasty little show right in front of our plate!

After a gorgeous dinner with all the trimmings, we knew a party would follow. I was feeling overfed from such a big meal, and tired, and not particularly interested in sex. Besides, I had no idea what the game plan was. It was hard to get excited with no expectation of what might happen. We went upstairs to change clothes. "Into what?" I wondered. What was the theme? I'd always heard that the costume makes the character, so I dived into my costume and toy bag. I needed a serious jolt of energy; nothing soft and flowing would do it for me tonight. I strapped on my dildo harness, into which I had inserted a large, bright purple dildo. Then I shook my breasts into a leather cupless bra and picked up a riding crop. I had begun to wake up a little. I would fake it till I felt sexy. Then I gave myself permission to sit back and watch if that was all I wanted to do. The minute I did so, I felt energized. I set off in search of some action to match my hard-edged mood.

Still not all that sure of myself, I cruised down the stairs to the living room, following the sound of Janis Joplin's "Piece of My Heart." Betty, dressed in leather chaps, stood behind Patricia, teasing her with a huge strap-on dildo. Patricia was also dressed in leather, though her outfit wasn't much more than a few straps. Before I could ask if I could join them, they said, "*Ooo*, you look hot; come on over here." Encouraged, I made my way over to Betty and stood behind her. I did to her whatever she did to Patricia. The scene melted its way into a three-way fuck, suck, bite, and wrestlefest that lasted considerably longer than the Joplin album.

When the three of us had recovered, I was dispatched to find out what everyone else was up to. I made my way upstairs, where I heard giggling from the bathroom off the master bedroom. Lost in the pleasures of a bathtub filled with rose-smelling bubbles and sweet, wet flesh, our three friends caressed, licked, and fingered each other. When they saw me—still sporting my leather and dildo—they decided it was time for the water goddesses to join the leather goddesses on the living room floor.

Downstairs, we all formed a circle, lying on our backs with knees up and vibrators in hand. Someone put a Springsteen album on the stereo. Using the conscious rhythmic breathing, the Kegels, and the vibrator techniques we had all mastered in Betty's workshops, we wove the hard and soft energies with which we had been playing into the most powerful jill-off I have ever been a part of. I came over and over again for twenty-five minutes—until I finally managed to stagger outside. I threw myself down on the cool, wet grass. I had left my vibrator inside the house and I was just lying on my back, but I was still coming. The earth rose up to meet me and the stars danced on my breasts and belly. I felt like an invincible bridge between the earthly and the mystical, filled with pure divine power.

The next morning we met in our circle with our coffee, sharing what had happened for us, each of us grateful and amazed at how powerful and life-changing sex could be among the right friends.

The Dark Heart

Chester Mainard and I created the Dark Heart ritual for the Great Australian Bliss Out and Love In. It was an evening in the middle of an intensive five-day residential workshop. The evening was called Dark Heart in reference to the many dark emotions and hurt feelings that had arisen out of a previous workshop exercise, during which some participants found themselves recreating old, destructive patterns of sexual behavior. The Dark Heart was designed to be a play space in which participants had the freedom to create the sexual experience they wanted and also to provide an environment with rules that supported conscious behavior. It was a space in which the dark and wounded heart could be embraced, honored, and healed with attention, love, and consciousness.

Chester transformed our usually light, airy, sun-filled workshop room into a cushioned, womblike, tomblike space. He had placed a few candles around the room, and a ray of soft moonlight filtered in through one window. That was the only light. The room was divided into four areas. Each area was set aside for a specific activity, and only for that activity.

The first area was for communicating. If you wanted to talk with someone and you were not being sexual at that time, you sat in the communication area. There you could negotiate what you and your partner wanted to do or share something about what you had done. You could also sit in this area if you were waiting to talk to someone. The only talking permitted in the other areas was necessary communication directly relating to the activity at hand.

The second area was for selfloving. Here you could masturbate alone or with others. You could also sit in this space if you simply wanted to be alone or meditate.

The other two spaces were for sexual or sensual interactions. Both had massage tables. One area was for people working in pairs, the other for people working in groups of more than two. At different times during the evening, one area was used for sensual massage while the other was used for erotic massage and actual lovemaking.

In order to move from, say, selfloving to a partner or group activity, you had to leave the selfloving area and move to the communication area to discuss what you wanted to do. Then you would move to the appropriate play space. If anyone attempted a conversation outside the communication area, they were gently escorted there. Similarly, if you wanted to join someone in the selfloving area for erotic touch, you had to leave the selfloving area and move to the appropriate space.

We were all a bit worried that this would end up as a whole lot of regimentation with no purpose or pleasure in it. In fact, the ritual was as hot as it was fascinating. We all learned how easy it is to slip into unconsciousness, and how equally easy it is to go back into being conscious. The Dark Heart was a ritual with consciousness built into its design and its rules. It allowed for our changes of moods, minds, and hearts; it only asked that we be aware of those changes. Because we could see and hear what was happening in the other areas of the room, the energy from each area fed into the others, which was intensely erotic. Each of us could be alone while feeling that we could come together easily. Dark Heart followed a day in which we had gone from pleasure to pleasure to way over the pleasure line into the unpleasant realization that we had recreated the sexual excesses of our past. It was a perfect way to deal with the stresses we were feeling. We came together erotically in spite of them.

If you have ever been curious but a little shy about trying sex in groups, I hope you're now feeling more inspired and encouraged. If you're a longtime group sex ritual lover, you've now got some more ideas to incorporate into your own rituals. Finally, if you and your partner would like to experiment with some group play but are feeling apprehensive about its impact on your relationship, you'll find a few guidelines on the following pages that I hope will help. Play safe and have fun!

How to Try Group Sex without Fracturing Your Relationship

1. The single most important rule to expanding your erotic life beyond your primary relationship is this: you must be completely honest, honorable, reliable, and trustworthy about the agreements you make when you try group sex, or any other kind of polyamory. If you aren't prepared to tell the truth, behave with integrity, and keep your promises, it won't work out, so you needn't read any further.

2. Discuss with your partner what specifically interests you about group sex. What delights you? What terrifies you? What would you like to discover for (or about) yourself in the experience? Is your partner interested in exploring it as well? What would they like out of it? If they are not interested, would they be open to your trying it alone? Under what, if any, circumstances would it be okay with them? (Perhaps a workshop would be okay, but a private party would not.)

3. What kind of erotic play do you each want to explore? If you want to explore Tantra and your partner wants to explore BDSM, it's likely you'll need to go to different events to get your needs met. Will you accompany each other to events or attend different events (on the same night or different nights)?

4. Decide what size and type of group would best serve your needs. A small workshop? A large play party? A medium-sized swingers' evening? Would you prefer to go to a couples-only event, or not?

5. Make mutually agreed-upon rules for yourselves. Which activities are you comfortable with and which are you not? For instance, you and your partner may decide that you'd love to have sex in a group setting, but only with each other. If you and your partner are comfortable being sexual with others, set limits. For example, perhaps it's fine with you if your partner gives someone a hand job, but not a blow job. Your partner may be comfortable with you participating in a BDSM scene so long as there is no genital contact. Perhaps all lower chakra penetrative sex is off limits, but oral sex is not. Whatever your rules, follow them scrupulously! If you find them too restrictive, don't break them and then tell your partner; follow them and then discuss modifying them with your partner later.

6. Set time limits. Agree on how long you are willing to be apart or engaged with someone else; tell your new partners at the beginning of your encounter and set the timer on your watch. If you and your partner attend separate events, or if one of

you is attending an event without the other, agree on a time and place to meet after the event, and be there on time.

7. Go slowly. Give yourselves time to discover your limits and your needs. If either you or your partner is feeling hurt or uncomfortable, it's time to create a new rule.

8. Make sure both you and your partner are getting your needs met. Ask yourself, "What is best for me, my partner, and my relationship?" If you fancy someone and want to play one-on-one with them, but it makes your partner uncomfortable, then, obviously, playing with them would not be best for your partner or your relationship. Don't do it. On the other hand, if you want to go to a sex workshop that you feel is important for your personal self-development and your partner feels threatened, you may decide that you will attend the workshop anyway. If you have demonstrated that you are honest, honorable, reliable, and trustworthy in your other agreements around sex and groups, it is likely that your partner will be able to accept your decision.

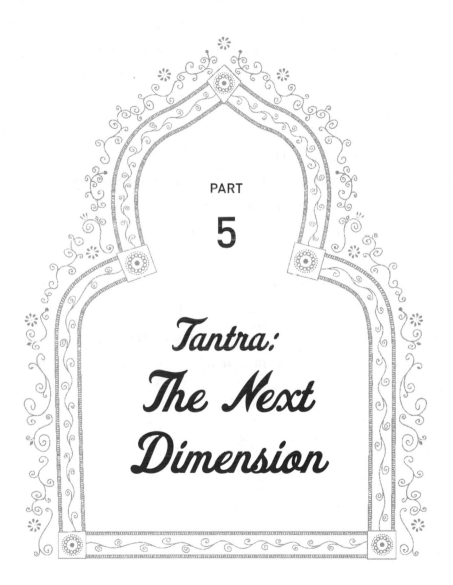

PART

5

Tantra: The Next Dimension

The possibilities of sex and sexual expression are infinite. If you have begun to practice Tantra you'll probably have noticed that your concept of what sex is and what you can do with it has expanded significantly. Now you're ready for the next step. It's time to take sex past the boundaries of pleasure and even of expanded consciousness and spiritual growth. It's time to enter the realm of sex magic.

I first discovered Tantra and sex magic when I needed practical and spiritual tools to help me cope with the illness and death of dozens of friends in the AIDS crisis. Not surprisingly, I first used sex magic for healing. This is still my primary use for sex magic, although over the years I have expanded my definition of healing to include not only personal but also social and political issues. I have even used sex magic to help me understand and accept death.

In this section of the book you'll see how you can use sex and sexual energy to heal yourself and to help others heal. You'll learn how to say "sexual prayers" for people, places, and causes you wish to support. Most of all, you'll learn how the art of sex magic can transform your relationship to your community, your world, and All That Is.

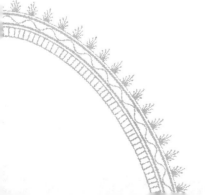

CHAPTER 22

Sex Magic

According to the Tarot, magic is the art of transformation. We have been practicing sex magic since page one. There is nothing all that magical about sex magic. It's as logical and often as predictable as technology. A century ago, it was magical that a voice could be transmitted through a telephone wire. Fifteen years ago, it seemed equally magical that a signal could be transmitted from one mobile phone to another without wires. Sex magic also comes in wired or wireless. The hardwired aspect of sex magic is the mind/body connection.

You experienced that when you focused all your attention on to one little finger in the Focused Awareness exercise (see chapter 2). Remember how that finger became more sensitive and alive than your other fingers? That's an excellent example of a hardwired mind/body connection that seems like magic. But what about wireless sex magic? What about the other day when you thought of someone you hadn't heard from for years and they called you the very next day? Is that a coincidence? Is it magic? Or might that be an example of some kind of wireless connection between you and that other person?

Sex magic can be as simple and as wired as masturbating to relax or to fall asleep. Sex magic can be as unwired as sending an orgasm as a prayer to promote peace in the Middle East. For people who believe in a higher power and talk with or pray to that higher power, sex magic may seem either logical or heretical, depending on the nature of your beliefs. Sex magic has a lot in common with prayer; we do conscious sex magic to accomplish any or all of several intentions:

* To connect with a higher power
* To send healing energy
* To influence the outcome of a given situation

What else might you do with the sexual energy you raise?

Sex magic is what happens when you put your sexual energy where your intentions are. Dedicated sex magicians feel that the earth is their church and their body is their altar as they dedicate their sexual energy for the benefit of themselves, their community, and their world. Sex magic is not religion, although it can certainly feel like a physical prayer. It is not Paganism, although it can be included in Pagan or Wiccan rituals. It is not at odds with any spiritual practice. It can be practiced within the structures of most nonfundamentalist religions. What makes sex magic different from other types of magic or prayer is the sheer power of the erotic. When you are in a high state of sexual excitement, enormous quantities of energy are released in the body, producing a trancelike state of consciousness. When you are in this hypnotic state of sexual excitement, you become especially receptive and impressionable. Visions you hold—and words you hear—at this time are powerfully imprinted on your consciousness. (This is why partners need to be especially aware of what they say to each other during lovemaking.) This combination of energy and receptivity offers a unique opportunity for transformation.

Sex and Healing

A few years ago, an article that appeared in the health section of the *New York Times* reported the less-than-astonishing news that a scientific study revealed that positive experiences can significantly boost the immune system, while negative events were shown to suppress it. This was reported as though millions of people had not already discovered this. There was one interesting twist to the study. The boost to the immune system that results from pleasant events can last as long as two days, while the negative effects of a stressful encounter mainly take their toll in just one day. So finally, there it was in print in the *New York Times*: a scientific study that clearly demonstrated that pleasure is more powerful than pain. Yet it is remarkable how rarely pleasure is ever mentioned as a tool when dealing with disease, illness, and pain.

I once observed a terminally ill cancer patient feel tremendously better after a half hour of watching Annie Sprinkle's sexually explicit one-woman show on tape. Color came into her face, she was more alive, and she was suddenly interested in having a little something to eat. No, she wasn't interested in having sex with anyone. That's not the point. Using our sexual energy as healing energy does not necessarily mean being turned on erotically or being interested in having sex with a partner. Our sexual energy is our life-force energy. When we activate it, we can use it for our healing and empowerment.

My brother Bill once drove across the state of Florida to be with his lover, Drew, who was then in the hospital. They were both in the late stages of AIDS. Bill called me from the car phone, sounding so terrible, so desperately ill, I didn't think he was going to make it to the hospital in Ft. Lauderdale. I felt completely helpless. As we spoke, one of my guardian angels whispered in my ear, "Tell him to stop at a gas station and cruise some guys." I thought that was pretty weird, but I couldn't think of anything else to say, so I said, "Bill, why don't you do what we always used to do when the drive was long and boring. Pull into a gas station, stand around, and cruise some guys." Bill said dispiritedly, "Oh yeah right. Those days are long gone." He was on so many body-numbing drugs that he hadn't felt sexual for months, if not years. But I kept trying. I teased him by saying, "You know those hunky guys in the tank tops with the gorgeous biceps that quiver when they pump the gas . . . the ones with the suntans and the blonde hair and the cute little buns?" After a few minutes of that kind of banter, he finally laughed and said, "Look, there's a gas station up ahead. I think I am going to stop." He sounded like the healthy Bill I used to know years before. That little shot of sexual energy got him across the entire state of Florida.

You can use your sexual energy for your own health and well-being. Let's look at some examples of the healing power of sex that you may already be familiar with and some that might surprise you.

Using Sex Magic to Relax and Relieve Stress

How many times have you had sex—with a partner or with yourself—and then gone straight to sleep? How many times have you masturbated in order to relax and be able to go to sleep? Wilhelm Reich, the revolutionary sex researcher, made the study of orgasm as a vital healing force his life's work. What Reich found in his scientific studies wasn't so different from what had been discovered centuries before in Asia. Reich claimed that orgone energy (which other traditions call Kundalini or chi) streams up and down the body from the top of the head to the bottom of the feet and back again. This energy is built up by taking in food, water, and air and is subsequently discharged by normal human activities such as emotional expression, the thinking process, body heat and growth, and excretion. In the normal course of one's life, more energy is built up than is discharged. This buildup of energy creates a tension—even without the stresses we experience in today's modern life. The most reliable method that nature has created for the release of that tension is sexual orgasm.

You may have noticed that a headache will go away if you masturbate and lie quietly for a few moments. You've breathed more deeply and opened up your blood vessels.

Oxygenated blood went to your brain. Endorphins were released. By the time you stood up, the headache wasn't so bad or it was just plain gone. If you haven't experienced this, try it. The same is true for menstrual cramps. Just when you think that sex is the last thing you are interested in, get out the vibrator. The sexual energy you generate opens up and relaxes the entire pelvic area. This will work almost all the time. If it doesn't wipe out all your cramps, it will reduce them considerably.

Using Sex Magic to Relieve Colds and Sinus Pain

Sex can open up your sinus passages and make the symptoms of a cold much less severe. What's more, sex is a lot more fun than popping mind-numbing antihistamines, which increase your blood pressure and add even more tension to an already tense you. One time as I was flying from New York to Australia, I had a bad cold. When I got off the plane, my head was pounding, my sinuses were sealed shut, and I was miserably jet-lagged. When I finally settled into my room, I lay down and turned on my vibrator. I gave myself an orgasm—not a particularly mind-blowing one, just a nice one. I meditated for about fifteen minutes, and when I got up, I could breathe clearly for the first time in sixteen hours. My headache was gone and I felt oriented enough in time and space to be able to participate in the day.

Sex brings us back to our own body rhythm. It takes us home, both physically and psychically. Using sex for self-healing does not have to include partner sex. Often, when we are not feeling well, the last thing we are interested in is sex with a partner; we just don't have the energy to give to someone else. You can masturbate or you can simply receive from your partner. Either way, the raising and releasing of sexual energy brings you back to yourself and nurtures your body. Like magic.

Using Sex Magic to Relieve Pain and Fear

Sex releases endorphins, those friendly little feel-good brain chemicals that are powerful enough to lift us out of pain and into euphoria. Some years ago, I had a little cyst in the middle of my back. I'm very sensitive in the solar plexus/third chakra, so I'm not very open to the idea of surgery in that area. I went to a traditional medical doctor to have the cyst removed. While he was giving me a local anesthetic, he quizzed me about my favorite movies, what I did for a living, and what I thought of the weather. He had obviously learned in medical school that you should engage the patient in conversation at moments like this to distract them from what you are doing to them. But this chit chat was making me more and more anxious. I was getting nauseous. I asked him to please stop talking. I started to do some circular breathing, some visualization, and some Kegels.

Taking slow, easy, full breaths, I began to circulate sexual energy around my body in the Microcosmic Orbit. Within a minute or two, I felt as though I had partially left my body, especially the part the doctor was operating on. I was somewhat aware of what was going on, but I had transcended the fear and nausea. In fact, I was having a pretty good time! The poor doctor. He had never seen anything like this in his office before. He was a good sport about it, though. Some doctors simply can't cope when you mix sexual healing techniques with traditional medicine. One doctor told me that he would not treat me if I continued to do "that strange breathing" and make "those strange sounds." I found another doctor quite easily.

Using sexual energy as a pain reliever and relaxation tool can come in quite handy at the dentist. The trick is to move sexual energy around your body in such a way as not to interrupt the dentist's work. I usually use a slow Circular Breath and circulate energy from my pussy to my heart. I found myself a Zen Buddhist periodontist who'd also studied a lot of Kundalini yoga and some Tantra. There are quite a few Western medical practitioners who are closet Tantrikas. As this more enlightened dentist worked on my teeth, I listened to didgeridoo music, breathed, and did Kegels. This didn't require a lot of movement. I easily kept my upper body totally still while I let my pelvis slowly rock back and forth in rhythm with the Kegels and the breath. It's more like moving within your body rather than actually moving your body. I got through a entire mouthful of periodontal surgery feeling well and happy; and my dentist was impressed at how fast my gums healed. Experiment with this the next time you go to the dentist. Going to the dentist can bring up so much fear. The breathing will relax you; and when you concentrate on moving your sexual energy throughout your body, the combination of breath and subtle movement will take your focus off what's happening in your mouth. Remember, sex feels good because it produces endorphins, which we want more of when something hurts or upsets us.

Using Sex Magic to Facilitate Childbirth

In her book *Woman's Experience of Sex*, Sheila Kitzinger observes that birth today is treated as though it is a medical/surgical crisis. The mother feels imprisoned in a situation outside her control. Childbirth classes, including Lamaze, teach a breath that encourages a "hold it . . . push . . . shoot" style of giving birth that is more like the way men ejaculate than the way women orgasm. A woman is supposed to carry on holding, pushing, and shooting as long as she can, and then fall back exhausted.

The energy flowing through the body in childbirth—the pressure of contracting muscles, the downward movement of the baby, and the opening of soft tissues—can be powerfully erotic when a woman does what comes naturally. When a woman does what comes naturally, she will breathe in a pattern that corresponds almost exactly with that of sexual excitement and orgasm. Her breath will quicken as she builds up to an orgasm, or contraction. Her breath then slows down after an orgasm or contraction. Then the quickening of breath picks up again in preparation for the next orgasm or contraction, and so on.

Women who are about to give birth would be wise to take stock of what their bodies are doing when they have their best orgasms. Use that as the model on which to base the breathing, the movement, the peaking, and the resting of labor. If you are multiorgasmic, take note of the period of time between one orgasm and the next. Learn to fully appreciate the valleys between the orgasms. How do you build up the energy again for another orgasm? Apply the same consciousness to childbirth as you learned in sex. If you are not yet multiorgasmic, it might help to learn how to be before you give birth.

Women who have given birth before and after participating in my Erotic Awakening workshops have reported that their postworkshop labors were much easier. The breathing they had learned in order to move sexual energy was exactly the breathing they needed to use in labor.

Using Sex Magic to Alleviate Back Pain

Our spine is literally our support system, so it follows that back pain has a lot to do with support and survival. Caroline Myss, author of *Anatomy of the Spirit*, maintains that lower back pain is always related to finances or financial relationships, whether those relationships are of an intimate or business nature. And remember your chakras. The lower back is also part of the sexual energy center of the body. The fears that manifest as pain in this area can range from "Can I earn a living?" to "Can I find a partner?" and "Can I take care of myself?" Essentially, the issues of support and survival here boil down to trusting and receiving—the same issues that arise around sexuality.

Many of us have grown up with a belief that we need to struggle in order to survive, or that pleasure is something that we have to earn—we have to do something (usually something difficult) in order to have the right to enjoy ourselves. Learning to receive sexual pleasure can help us break out of this puritanical equation. When you both ask for pleasure and really receive it, you begin to reprogram your body and your mind, and you open yourself up to greater trust and the enjoyment of abundance, as well as a greater spirit of guilt-free generosity.

The next time you experience lower back pain, use sex as a physical affirmation. Visualize your sexual energy flowing up from your root chakra. Feel it opening up all your energy channels. Feel it expanding your energy field so that you can reach out and accept abundance and prosperity. You can say an affirmation such as, "I am open to receive all good" as you orgasm. The expansion and the power that results from this will center you and restore your trust in the natural flow of universal abundance. As a side benefit, your back will begin to feel a whole lot better.

Using Sex Magic to Heal Sexual Wounds

One of the most challenging issues we face when we talk about sexual healing lies in the area of sexual abuse. Sexual abuse wounds the body, the mind, and the emotions. Abuse most often occurs at times in our lives when we are particularly vulnerable. The wounds of sexual abuse are so deep and so profound, it's easy to feel that the spirit itself is wounded. Higher self/spirit cannot be wounded. The spirit is always intact. It's always whole and strong and particularly available to help us in a method of healing, which for lack of any other name, I call homeopathic sexuality.

Homeopathy is the branch of healing that uses "the hair of the dog" to cure the dog bite. No, we are absolutely not going to subject someone with a history of sexual abuse to even the smallest bit of more abuse. But we can use just the right amount and kind of sexual energy. Homeopathic sexuality is based on the understanding that our higher power can and will guide us to ways to work with our own sexual energy in order to heal past sexual traumas.

Forms of sexual abuse range from years of intense physical and emotional trauma to the less obvious varieties that nearly everyone has experienced: being humiliated for masturbating or for not fitting into the right gender mold, being coerced into having sex when you didn't want it, or being told you look like a whore when you're sixteen and have just spent two hours making yourself look beautiful for a date. The wounds may not be physical, but in this puritanical culture we are constantly wounded or abused emotionally as we grow up learning to be sexual. Whatever the physical or emotional circumstances, sexual abuse is abuse of power. Period.

Psychotherapist Dean Allen works extensively with energy medicine and the physical disorders created in the body by emotional traumas. He defines power as "the ability to meet pressure with pressure in such a way as to hold the outside force at bay, confront the issue with courage, and resolve the issue with pride." In cases of sexual abuse, the abused is in a situation where they are not able—or feel they are not able—to hold the abuser at bay. Once the abuse starts, they are not able to confront the issue, and they are certainly not able to resolve the issue with any pride. The abuser may be a parent or someone in authority; they may be larger and stronger.

The abuser's misuse of power is rooted in insecurity. Abusers have a win/lose mentality. According to Dean Allen, abusers believe that the source of their power is winning and that winning means overpowering someone else. Once begun, patterns of abuse often carry on for years and years, not to mention from generation to generation. The experience creates a debilitating drag on the energy of the sexual power center. Once in place, this drag will remain on the sexual energy center until the true power inherent in that center is restored through healing.

Healing sexual abuse through sexuality begins by peeling away the layers of armor we have built up to protect ourselves from further abuse. What does some of this armoring look like? It often manifests as hatred of the body and an extremely negative body image. That can range from putting on lots of weight (representing layers of protection) to anorexia and bulimia, which are attempts to make the body invisible. Armor may be in the form of sexual shutdown—loss of feeling in the sex organs and the inability to receive pleasure from sex. Armor can manifest as lack of boundaries or compulsive sex—the inability to say no to sex or the desire to seek it out in excess even though the person receives little or no pleasure from it. It's also very common for survivors of sexual abuse to experience real pleasure only when they are giving or receiving pain. (This is certainly not to say that everyone who loves BDSM is a survivor of sexual abuse.)

When the power in the sexual energy center has been drained, blocked, or dragged down, we seek to replace that power by attaching ourselves to situations or people that seem more powerful than we are. Later in life, we often look to exactly the same type of person as the first abuser.

Homeopathic sexuality is a gentle process that seeks to stimulate the body's natural healing response. In the case of sexual abuse, it means gently introducing the recovering person to the beauty and power of his or her own sexuality. Homeopathic sexuality is the step-by-step process of relearning pleasure. We move from sex as survival to sex as pleasure.

At first, any sort of invocation of sexual healing energy might be uncomfortable. As the sexual energy begins to peel away the armor, the layers of feeling underneath are very sensitive, very tender. As we gently move out beyond the protection of these layers, we find safety and empowerment. This can come in the form of being given a safe space and the permission to say no, thereby reestablishing more naturally healthy boundaries. Participating in a sexual healing workshop, where you are given the opportunity to say, "No, I really don't want to be touched right now," and have that wish honored and supported, can be worth a year in therapy. The discovery or rediscovery of what actually feels good, what feels bad, and what has no feeling at all—that's what I mean by a relearning.

I am not advocating any one path of sexual healing for sexual abuse. I am advocating some form of sexual healing. I have known people who have been in therapy for years and are still victims of their childhood sexual abuse; I have known others who are long-term survivors. The choice is up to each individual. Tantra can give you the time and space to experience your sexuality as a gift rather than as a wound. With its emphasis on consciousness and its support for a wide range of emotional and sexual expressions, Tantra can help heal past traumas and open up new avenues of trust and pleasure.

Sex Magic and Compulsive Sex

It is not the amount or type of sex someone has that determines sexually compulsive behavior, what the media is fond of calling "sex addiction"; rather, it's the obsession with having sex at the expense of most everything else. People living with this compulsion describe their need for sex the way people addicted to physical substances describe their needs. They feel out of control, unable to stop, obsessed with an elusive physical high they believe comes from sex. Sexual compulsives don't get high from the sex—they get high from the power. One woman described this as the power of getting someone to want her, to give her attention. It was about the chase, not the sex. The sex was the least of it—she said she felt empty afterward and wanted to get away as fast as she could. Sexual compulsives may even put themselves in real physical danger, because surviving that danger increases their feeling of power and, therefore, the high; it's an adrenaline rush. Not surprisingly, many sexual compulsives were sexually abused as children. They seek to restore the power that has been drained, blocked, or dragged down in their sexual energy centers by putting themselves in situations that make them feel powerful in relation to sex.

Sexual compulsion is often treated the way alcoholism or drug addiction is treated—by strict abstinence from sex. But sex is not like alcohol or drugs. It's more like breath and food. According to Taoist philosophy, the triple generators of life are food, breath, and sex. So completely shutting down one's sexuality during the recovery period is like saying, "I am powerless over food so I will never eat again" or "I caught a virus from breathing so I will never breathe again." We need to make the distinction between sexual activity and sexual energy. Certainly, abstaining from some forms of sexual activity can be a healthy choice—in the case of sexual compulsives and in many other cases. But that does not mean shutting down our sexual energy.

The more conscious we become of our sexual power, the more we are able to use it as a force for healing, for loving, for creativity, and for right action. Tantra and sex magic offer us the opportunity for personal and planetary transformation. When we are conscious of ourselves as alive, loving, erotic beings, we walk in the world with a greater awareness. We are appreciative of everyone else's alive, loving eroticism. We are more able to put ourselves in someone else's shoes. We stop feeling so separate.

Sex Magic in the Workplace

Instead of less sex in the workplace, I think we need more. More conscious use of sexual energy, that is. Despite all the laws against sexual harassment in the workplace, it doesn't seem to be going away. Why? Anything repressed will express itself in its darker form. So, a law saying "sexual expression of any kind is inappropriate in the workplace" sets up that workplace for rampant inappropriate displays of sexual expression. Instead of a ban on sexual expression, I'd like to see workplace seminars on the conscious use of sex in business.

Sex magic in the workplace does not involve intimate contact with the nearest sexually desirable person. My friend Marcy worked from home doing phone sales. Most of the people to whom she sold were men. She told me that whenever she sensed that a sale was slipping away, she would start doing Kegels as she continued her pitch. She reported that eighty to ninety percent of the time, the call turned around and she made the sale. Unwired sex magic strikes again!

Instead of repressing your sexuality in your workplace, how can you use your sexuality to help you accomplish your goals? Whether your workplace sex magic is wired or unwired, your conscious use of sexual energy will not only help you be more effective in your job, but it will also make your job a lot more pleasurable. On your way to work tomorrow, send some sex magic ahead of you. Do some circular breathing and start an erotic fantasy to get your sexual energy running. Kegel that energy up your body, out your heart center, and into your day. You can even imagine it landing on your boss's desk and coming back to you in the form of a raise. A few moments of sex magic on your way to work can help make your highest hopes a reality. As Annie Sprinkle is fond of saying, "If you make love to the Universe, the Universe makes love to you."

Sex Magic for World Peace, Part 1

Any Tantric ritual—solo, partner, or group—can become a healing ritual when it is performed on behalf of someone else, be they across the room, across town, or across the ocean. Years ago, Louise Hay taught me the technique of sending love to people and places that needed healing. As I learned more, I began sending orgasmic energy as well.

I dedicated orgasmic energy to ending apartheid in South Africa. I sent love and orgasms for years. Maybe the orgasms helped, maybe not. But every time I sent the people of South Africa an orgasm, I was reminded of the healing that was needed there. There is nothing like being erotically focused on something to make you more aware of it. I paid more attention to what was going on there; I sent money; I did whatever I could to support my sexual prayers.

Wouldn't it be wonderful if we could focus some of our excess sexual energy on healing the planet instead of focusing on personal romantic dramas that bring us pain? We each possess an unlimited amount of sexual energy. Each of us has enough to support a deeply intimate relationship plus enough to keep us healthy, happy, and whole. On top of that, we each have more than enough sexual energy left over to donate to the healing of someone else.

You have learned many ways to circulate sexual energy within yourself, with a partner, or throughout a group. Now let's expand that. Pick one of your favorite Tantric techniques or visualizations. Pick a place in the world that could use some healing. Now adapt the exercise you chose so that you direct as much love and bliss to that place as you would normally give to yourself or to a partner. You can send your sexual energy to a country or to a group of people or to just one person in need of spiritual, emotional, or physical help.

Before you begin, state your intention. Make it as inclusive and as open as possible. For example, if I want to send sex magic/healing to the Tibetan people living in exile or under the yoke of Chinese dictatorship, I may not know what kind of healing is actually required. Instead of saying, "I dedicate my sexual energy to anything that gets the Chinese out of Tibet," I would say, "I dedicate my sexual energy as a physical prayer for peace and healing for the people of Tibet. May this healing occur in whatever form is in the highest good for the people of Tibet and for all concerned."

Don't be afraid to ask for outside help. Call in spirit helpers on behalf of your beneficiary. Spirit helpers include gods, goddesses, angels, devas, fairies, and so on. Call both your own spirit helpers as well as those of your beneficiaries. Ask that your sexual energy join all the energy in the Universe that also desires healing for your person or country or situation.

Think universally, fuck locally!

After you have made your dedication, let go of it. Trust that your intention is manifesting at exactly the right time, in exactly the right place, and in exactly the perfect manner. You do not need to focus on it at every moment during your sex magic ritual. If you did, you wouldn't be conscious and present in your ritual. Do what you would do in any Tantric ritual—focus on the sexual energy. I like to return to the thought of my dedication just before or just after the moment of orgasm. I like to visualize or feel my intention becoming manifest. This is my personal choice and may not be right for everyone.

Dedicating your orgasms to include a purpose beyond your own pleasure will remind you that your sexuality is a sacred and a powerful tool of transformation. You can dedicate your orgasms and/or sexual energy as a prayer for a wide variety of reasons, such as the following:

* You can ask for wisdom about work, school, or a relationship, or for help in making a decision.
* You can send orgasmic energy to help heal a friend's illness, the AIDS crisis in Africa, your own depression, and so on.
* You can dedicate an orgasm to someone in gratitude for the help they gave you, to your parents on their anniversary, or to a world leader who is working on behalf of peace and justice. Better yet, dedicate an orgasm to a world leader you do *not* feel is doing the right thing.
* You can simply dedicate your orgasm to your own highest good and for the highest good of everyone on the planet.

Sex Magic for World Peace, Part 2

I practice a powerful meditation I learned from the Dalai Lama. It is a Tibetan Buddhist meditation called Tonglen. In Tonglen, you breathe in all the pain and suffering of the world and breathe out peace, prosperity, and happiness.

Breathe the suffering of the world into your heart and breathe out happiness, bliss for all beings.
   When you inhale, take upon yourself the suffering of other sentient beings. Then when you exhale, give your prosperity, your virtues, your happiness to all sentient beings.
                                                                    —His Holiness, the Dalai Lama

Tonglen is a method for awakening the compassion inherent in all of us. The Dalai Lama points out that whatever suffering exists in the world comes from cherishing one's own interest; whatever happiness exists comes from cherishing the welfare of others. Tonglen is a method for overcoming our fear of suffering and for dissolving the tightness of our heart, both of which conditions arise from cherishing ourselves over others.

Tonglen can be a particularly powerful form of sex magic. Instead of breathing into and out of my heart, I breathe into my pussy and out my heart, or into my heart and out my pussy. I activate my Kundalini energy to connect with and help alleviate the suffering of all those who I feel are in great need of healing, especially those suffering from sexual abuse and sexual violence.

Tonglen is not some airy-fairy visualization. You really send your happiness out. You really take on the suffering of others. Tonglen is very powerful; you may want to start small. You could begin the practice by taking on the suffering of one person you know to be hurting—someone you wish to help. For example, if you know of a child who is hurting, you breathe in all the pain and fear of that child. On the wings of your outgoing breath, you send the child happiness, joy, or whatever might relieve their pain.

Once you're comfortable with performing Tonglen for one person, increase the scope of your ritual. Perform your Tonglen for a family, a neighborhood, a region, a nation, a continent, and the planet itself, keeping in mind that you are quite literally breathing in the pain and suffering of people, not the abstract idea of pain and suffering. Move outward slowly and pick your suffering carefully, particularly if you are doing my sex magic variation on the practice.

Tonglen may seem peculiarly masochistic, but I assure you it doesn't feel that way. Tonglen gives me a healthier perspective on the world. It makes me feel like I am helping people in some small way and that makes me feel stronger, more capable, and more connected to all the beings on the planet.

Try it. Breathe in for all of us and breathe out for all of us.

Sex and Death

You've probably heard or experienced for yourself that sexual arousal is one of the most common reactions to the death of a loved one. While many people feel ashamed of this reaction, from a Tantric perspective, the turn-on not only makes sense, it's totally natural for two very good reasons:

* The body knows it needs a powerful release of tension and emotion, so it wants sex.
* Death and grief make us feel lost and disconnected. Sex makes us feel alive and brings us back home to our bodies.

When it comes to death, sex and orgasm do more than relieve grief and pain. Orgasm is often referred to as "the little death." Similarly, death is sometimes called "the ultimate orgasm." Earlier in this book, I detailed my experience of leaving my body and visiting my dead friends during my first Erotic Awakening Massage. That experience taught me like nothing else the depth of the connection between death and orgasm. Letting go as completely as we can in orgasm is as close as we can get to death without actually dying. In the afterglow of an orgasm, you get a taste of what it is like to have your soul temporarily released from the earth trance, which your mind experiences as reality.

Ram Dass, author, teacher, and longtime spiritual seeker, had a massive stroke in 1997. He is now exploring the spiritual landscape of aging and dying. He calls death "ripening into God." His description of the meditations he is using to prepare for death sound very similar to what happens to us in orgasm:

When you deepen into a moment, you disappear—at least the solid "you" that you're used to experiencing disappears. Everything around you—maybe it's a palm tree, dripping water, cars honking, people racing past you—everything feels ecstatic when you free yourself into the moment. You recognize your interconnectedness, and all these things in a moment can become mystical doorways for the soul. In this state you can't worry about the past or the future and you can't worry about "me," because you can no longer find a separate "me." In the moment we become free from the Ego's desires and open to the Soul. We interrupt the Ego melodrama. The soap opera takes a break for a message from our sponsor: God.

The conscious use of orgasm to prepare for death may not answer questions like "What happens at the precise moment of death?" or "What happens after we die?" but I can tell you from personal experience that the conscious use of orgasm can alleviate much of our fear of death. At the risk of sounding macabre, I've come to love practicing death.

You need only be clear and committed in your intention to know something more of death. Given clarity of intention, you can perform a ritual/mediation with the consciousness you have developed thus far in Tantra. You are likely to have revealing, rewarding experiences. Keep in mind that the more sexual energy you raise, the more likely you are to have full, rich orgasmic experiences that leave you with the timeless, egoless, bodiless feeling of an after-death experience. Your practice of death is less about what you do than how you do it. You can use any and many Tantric techniques to raise this energy. The Erotic Awakening Massage ritual is a particularly effective path to this end. While you are designing your Erotic Awakening Massage ritual, keep the following principles in mind:

* Commit to your sexual pleasure, your sexual energy, and your orgasm.
* As you breathe, Kegel, fuck, or flog, visualize your intention to know death better.
* You may visualize briefly stepping out of your body, seeing yourself as spirit, or becoming peace or silence or a part of All That Is.
* You may visualize being embraced by God/dess or even kissing Death on the lips.
* At the point of orgasm, let go as completely as you can. Release your visualization. Let your body go, your mind go, your emotions go.
* Do nothing, plan nothing, be nothing. Let death happen to you in whatever form it chooses to take.
* Make no judgments about what happens.

My other favorite death meditation is energetically quite different. It is done with a partner. One of you will "die" and the other will witness the "death." If you are the one who is "dying," lie down flat on your back in the yoga corpse pose with your arms and legs extended and relaxed. Your partner sits on the floor next to you and just witnesses. The rest is simple: all you do is die. How do you die? Well, that's what you discover in the course of the meditation. Your breath may get shallow, you may have visions; everyone's method of death and experience of dying is different. And that's the point. There is no one way to die. You may find that dying is very easy for you; you may find it very difficult. That is also appropriate. This meditation is not about who dies better, faster, or more easily. It's about opening yourself up to a closer, healthier relationship with death.

If you are the witnessing partner in this meditation, try to keep your eyes open or partially open most of the time. Stay present with your partner. Even though you are only witnessing, keep in mind that witnessing death is in and of itself a powerful experience. As a witness, you too may experience visions; your partner's face may appear to change. You may feel emotional; it may bring up memories or visions or feelings about the death of a loved one. If you believe in past lives, you may even experience some of your own deaths.

It is said that only through death do we really know life. Each time you perform a death meditation, you are likely to discover a new aspect of death. Every time you embrace death a bit more tightly, your delight in life expands proportionately.

As I am sure you realize by now, Tantra is about far more than sex. In Tantra, all worldly activities are opportunities to experience the divine, especially when they are approached with consciousness and intention. Sex is simply one particularly delightful and powerful way to tap into the pleasures and desires that permeate the entire universe. As you dive totally into each present moment in sex, you tap into universal ecstasy. Soon you will be able to make that same ecstatic connection in other areas of your life. When you live Tantrically, you live with love and passion for all of life, and with a consistent, blissful connection to All That Is and All That You Are.

References

Albury, Kath. *Yes Means Yes: Getting Explicit about Heterosex.* Crows Nest, NSW, Australia: Allen & Unwin, 2002.

Alder, Dr. Harry. *Neuro Linguistic Programming: The Art and Science of Getting What You Want.* London: Judy Piatkus, 1994.

Allen, Marcus. *Tantra for the West: A Guide to Personal Freedom.* San Rafael, CA: New World Library, 1981.

Anand, Margo. *The Art of Sexual Ecstasy: The Path of Sacred Sexuality for Western Lovers.* Los Angeles: Jeremy P. Tarcher, 1989.

Anderson, Bruce. *Tantra for Gay Men.* Los Angeles: Alyson Publications, 2002.

Bornstein, Kate. *Gender Outlaw: On Men, Women, and the Rest of Us.* New York: Routledge, 1994.

———. *My Gender Workbook: How to Become a Real Man, a Real Woman, the Real You, or Something Else Entirely.* New York: Routledge, 1998.

Brame, Gloria G., William Brame, and Jon Jacobs. *Different Loving: The World of Sexual Dominance & Submission.* New York: Villard, 1993.

Brauer, Alan P., MD, and Donna J. Brauer. *ESO: How You and Your Lover Can Give Each Other Hours of Extended Sexual Orgasm.* New York: Warner Books, 1983.

Chia, Mantak, and Douglas Abrams Arava. *The Multi-Orgasmic Man: Sexual Secrets Every Man Should Know.* New York: HarperCollins, 1996.

Chia, Mantak, and Maneewan Chia. *Healing Love through the Tao: Cultivating Female Sexual Energy.* Huntington, NY: Healing Tao Books, 1986.

Chia, Mantak, Maneewan Chia, Douglas Abrams, and Rachel Abrams, MD. *The Multi-Orgasmic Couple: Sexual Secrets Every Couple Should Know.* New York: HarperCollins, 2000.

Chinmoy, Sri. *Kundalini: The Mother-Power.* Jamaica, NY: Agni Press, 1974.

Clow, Barbara Hand. *Liquid Light of Sex: Understanding Your Key Life Passages.* Rochester, VT: Bear & Company, 1996.

Dass, Ram. *Still Here: Embracing Aging, Changing, and Dying.* New York: Riverhead Books, 2000.

Dodson, Betty. *Orgasms for Two: The Joy of Partnersex.* New York: Harmony Books, 2002.

———. *Sex for One: The Joy of Selfloving.* New York: Crown Publishing Group, 1996.

Easton, Dossie, and Catherine Liszt. *The Topping Book: Or, Getting Good At Being Bad*. San Francisco: Greenery Press, 1995.

———. *The Bottoming Book: Or, How to Get Terrible Things Done to You by Wonderful People*. San Francisco: Greenery Press, 1994.

Feuerstein, Georg. *Enlightened Sexuality: Living the Vision of the Erotic Spirit*. Freedom, CA: Crossing Press, 1989.

———. *Sacred Sexuality: Living the Vision of the Erotic Spirit*. New York: Jeremy P. Tarcher/Perigee Books, 1993.

———. "Tantrism and Neotantrism." *Moksha Journal* (www.santosha.com/moksha/tantrism1 .html), 1996.

Garrison, Omar. *Tantra: The Yoga of Sex*. New York: Harmony Books, 1964.

Gay Men's Health Crisis. "Making Your Own Decisions, Frequently Asked Questions—and Some Answers—about Gay Sex." *GMHC* (www.gmhc.org), 1995–2002.

Geba, Bruno Hans. *Breathe Away Your Tension: An Introduction to Gestalt Body Awareness Therapy*. New York: Random House, 1977.

Gold, E. J., and Cybele Gold. *Tantric Sex*. Playa Del Rey, CA: Peak Skill Publishing, 1988.

Guy, David. *The Red Thread of Passion: Spirituality and the Paradox of Sex*. Boston, MA: Shambala Publications, 1999.

Hagen, Steve. *Buddhism Plain and Simple*. New York: Broadway Books, 1998.

Hanley, Jesse Lynn, MD, and Nancy Deville. *Tired of Being Tired*. New York: G. P. Putnam's Sons, 2001.

Hawkins, David R., MD. *Power vs. Force*. Carlsbad, CA: Hay House, 2002.

Hay, Louise L. *You Can Heal Your Life*. Carlsbad, CA: Hay House, 2004.

Henderson, Julie. *The Lover Within*. Barrytown, NY: Station Hill Press, 1987.

Henes, Donna. "On Being Prepared." *Always in Season: Living in Sync with the Cycle* 13 (Winter 2001).

Hutchins, Loraine. "Erotic Rites: A Cultural Analysis of Contemporary U.S. Sacred Sexuality Traditions and Trends." PhD diss., Union Institute Graduate College, 2001.

Joannides, Paul. *Guide to Getting It On!* Waldport, OR: Goofy Foot Press, 2000.

Johnson, Robert A. *Ecstasy: Understanding the Psychology of Joy*. San Francisco: HarperSanFrancisco, 1987.

———. *Owning Your Own Shadow: Understanding the Dark Side of the Psyche*. San Francisco: HarperSanFrancisco, 1991.

Jwala. *Sacred Sex: Ecstatic Techniques for Empowering Relationships*. San Rafael, CA: Mandala, 1993.

Kaufman, Miriam, MD, Cory Silverberg, and Fran Odette. *The Ultimate Guide to Sex and Disability*. San Francisco: Cleis Press, 2003.

Khalsa, Shakta Kaur. *K.I.S.S. Guide to Yoga*. New York: DK Publishing, 2001.

Kitzinger, Sheila. *Woman's Experience of Sex*. London: Penguin Books, 1983.

Lowen, Alexander, MD, and Leslie Lowen. *The Way to Vibrant Health: A Manual of Bioenergetic Exercises*. New York: Harper & Row, 1977.

Magee, Mike. "Sexuality in the Tantrik Tradition." *Shiva Shakti Mandalam* (www.shivashakti.com), 1995.

Montano, Linda M. "Chakra Prayers." *7 Years of Living Art + Another 7 Years of Living Art = 14 Years of Living Art* (www.bobsart.org/montano/living_art/index.html). 1984–1998.

Myss, Caroline, PhD. *Anatomy of the Spirit: The Seven Stages of Power and Healing*. New York: Harmony Books, 1996.

Newman, Felice. *The Whole Lesbian Sex Book*. San Francisco: Cleis Press, 2002.

Osho. *The Book of Secrets*. New York: St. Martin's Griffin, 1998.

———. *Meditation: The First and Last Freedom*. New York: St. Martin's Griffin, 1996.

———. *The Tantra Experience*. Poona, India: Rebel Publishing House, 1994.

———. *Tantric Transformation*. Poona, India: Rebel Publishing House, 1994.

Ramer, Andrew. *Two Flutes Playing: Spiritual Love/Sacred Sex*. Oakland, CA: Body Electric Publishing, 1990.

Ramsdale, David and Ellen. *Sexual Energy Ecstasy: A Practical Guide to Lovemaking Secrets of the East and West*. Playa Del Rey, CA: Peak Skill Publishing, 1991.

Reich, Wilhelm. *The Function of the Orgasm: Sex-Economic Problems of Biological Energy*. New York: Farrar, Strauss and Giroux, 1973.

Rush, Anne Kent. *Getting Clear: Body Work for Women*. New York: Random House, 1973; Berkeley, CA: Bookworks, 1973.

Schnarch, David, PhD. *Resurrecting Sex: Resolving Sexual Problems and Rejuvenating Your Relationship*. New York: HarperCollins, 2002.

Selby, John. *Peak Sexual Experience*. New York: Warner Books, 1992.

Semans, Anne, and Cathy Winks. *The Woman's Guide to Sex on the Web*. San Francisco: HarperSanFrancisco, 1999.

Sky, Michael. *Breathing: Expanding Your Power & Energy*. Santa Fe, NM: Bear & Company, 1990.

Society for Human Sexuality. "Guide to Safer Sex (Concise)." Society for Human Sexuality (www.sexuality.org/concise.html), 2002.

Sunyata, and Bodhi Avinasha. *Jewel in the Lotus: The Sexual Path to Higher Consciousness*. San Francisco: Kriya Jyoti Tantra Society, 1987.

Tannahill, Reay. *Sex in History*. Chelsea, MI: Scarborough House, 1992.

Tunneshende, Merilyn. *Don Juan and the Art of Sexual Energy: The Rainbow Serpent of the Toltecs*. Rochester, VT: Bear & Company, 2001.

Winks, Cathy, and Anne Semans. *The Good Vibrations Guide to Sex*. San Francisco: Cleis Press, 2002.

Woods, Margo. *Masturbation, Tantra and Self Love*. San Diego: Omphaloskepsis Press, 1981.

Resources

Books

BDSM

Deviant Desires: Incredibly Strange Sex, by Katherine Gates (Juno Books, 2000).

Different Loving: The World of Sexual Dominance & Submission, by Gloria G. Brame, William Brame, and Jon Jacobs (Villard, 1993).

The New Bottoming Book, by Dossie Easton and Janet W. Hardy (Greenery Press, 2003).

The New Topping Book, by Dossie Easton and Janet W. Hardy (Greenery Press, 2001).

Radical Ecstasy: SM Journeys to Transcendence, by Dossie Easton and Janet W. Hardy (Greenery Press, 2004).

SM 101: A Realistic Introduction, by Jay Wiseman (Greenery Press, 1998).

GLBTQ

Gender Outlaw: On Men, Women, and the Rest of Us, by Kate Bornstein (Routledge, 1994).

Miss Vera's Finishing School for Boys Who Want to Be Girls, by Veronica Vera (Main Street Books, 1997).

My Gender Workbook: How to Become a Real Man, a Real Woman, the Real You, or Something Else Entirely, by Kate Bornstein (Routledge, 1998).

Two Flutes Playing: Spiritual Love/Sacred Sex, by Andrew Ramer (Body Electric Publishing, 1990).

The Whole Lesbian Sex Book, by Felice Newman (Cleis Press, 2002).

MASSAGE

Erotic Massage: The Tantric Touch of Love, by Kenneth Ray Stubbs, PhD (Jeremy P. Tarcher, 1999).

Male Erotic Massage: A Guide to Sex and Spirit, by Kenneth Ray Stubbs, PhD, and Jim Dennis (Secret Garden Publishing, 1999).

MEDITATION

Living from the Heart: Heart Rhythm Meditation for Energy, Clarity, Peace, Joy, and Inner Power, by Puran Bair (Three Rivers Press, 1998).

Meditation: The First and Last Freedom, by Osho (St. Martin's Griffin, 1996).

MIND, BODY, AND SPIRIT

Anatomy of the Spirit: The Seven Stages of Power and Healing, by Caroline Myss, PhD (Harmony Books, 1996).

Breathing: Expanding Your Power & Energy, by Michael Sky (Bear & Company, 1990).

You Can Heal Your Life, by Louise L. Hay (Hay House, 2004).

SEX GUIDES AND HOW-TO BOOKS

Dr. Sprinkle's Spectacular Sex: Make Over Your Love Life with One of the World's Greatest Sex Experts, by Annie Sprinkle, PhD (Tarcher, 2005).

ESO: How You and Your Lover Can Give Each Other Hours of Extended Sexual Orgasm, by Alan P. Brauer, MD, and Donna J. Brauer (Warner Books, 1983).

The Ethical Slut: A Guide to Infinite Sexual Possibilities, by Dossie Easton and Catherine A. Liszt (Greenery Press, 1998).

Exhibitionism for the Shy, by Carol Queen (Down There Press, 1995).

The Good Vibrations Guide to Sex, by Cathy Winks and Anne Semans (Cleis Press, 2002).

Guide to Getting It On! by Paul Joannides (Goofy Foot Press, 2000).

How to Tell a Naked Man What to Do: Sex Advice from a Woman Who Knows, by Candida Royalle (Fireside, 2004).

Masturbation, Tantra and Self Love, by Margo Woods (Omphaloskepsis Press, 1981).

Orgasms for Two: The Joy of Partnersex, by Betty Dodson (Harmony Books, 2002).

Peak Sexual Experience, by John Selby (Warner Books, 1992).

Resurrecting Sex: Resolving Sexual Problems and Rejuvenating Your Relationship, by David Schnarch, PhD (HarperCollins, 2002).

Sex for One: The Joy of Selfloving, by Betty Dodson (Crown Publishing Group, 1996).

The Ultimate Guide to Sex and Disability, by Miriam Kaufman, MD, Cory Silverberg, and Fran Odette (Cleis Press, 2003).

The Western Guide to Feng Shui for Romance: The Dance of Heart and Home, by Terah Kathryn Collins (Hay House, 2004).

Woman's Experience of Sex, by Sheila Kitzinger (Penguin Books, 1983).

Yes Means Yes: Getting Explicit about Heterosex, by Kath Albury (Allen & Unwin, 2002).

TANTRA, TAO, AND SACRED SEX

The Art of Sexual Ecstasy: The Path of Sacred Sexuality for Western Lovers, by Margo Anand (Jeremy P. Tarcher, 1989).

The Book of Secrets, by Osho (St. Martin's Griffin, 1998).

The Complete Idiot's Guide to Tantric Sex, by Dr. Judy Kuriansky (Alpha Books, 2001).

Ecstasy Though Tantra, by Dr. Jonn Mumford (Llewellyn Publications, 1988).

Enlightened Sexuality: Living the Vision of the Erotic Spirit, by Georg Feuerstein (Crossing Press, 1989).

The Essence of Tantric Sexuality, by Mark A. Michaels and Patricia Johnson (Llewellyn Publications, 2006).

Healing Love through the Tao: Cultivating Female Sexual Energy, by Mantak Chia and Maneewan Chia (Healing Tao Books, 1986).

Jewel in the Lotus: The Sexual Path to Higher Consciousness, by Sunyata and Bodhi Avinasha (Kriya Jyoti Tantra Society, 1987).

The Lover Within, by Julie Henderson (Station Hill Press, 1987).

The Multi-Orgasmic Couple: Sexual Secrets Every Couple Should Know, by Mantak Chia, Maneewan Chia, Douglas Abrams, and Rachel Abrams, MD (HarperCollins, 2000).

The Multi-Orgasmic Man: Sexual Secrets Every Man Should Know, by Mantak Chia and Douglas Abrams Arava (HarperCollins, 1996).

The Multi-Orgasmic Woman: Discover Your Full Desire, Pleasure, and Vitality, by Mantak Chia and Rachel Abrams (Rodale Books, 2006).

The Red Thread of Passion: Spirituality and the Paradox of Sex, by David Guy (Shambala Publications, 1999).

Sacred Orgasms: Teachings of the Hearts, by Kenneth Ray Stubbs, PhD (Secret Garden Publishing, 1992).

Sacred Sex: Ecstatic Techniques for Empowering Relationships, by Jwala with Robb Smith (Mandala, 1993).

Sacred Sexuality: Living the Vision of the Erotic Spirit, by Georg Feuerstein (Jeremy P. Tarcher/ Perigee Books, 1993).

Sexual Energy Ecstasy: A Practical Guide to Lovemaking Secrets of the East and West, by David and Ellen Ramsdale (Peak Skill Publishing, 1991).

Sexual Secrets, by Nik Douglas and Penny Slinger (Inner Traditions International, 1999).

Tantra for Gay Men, by Bruce Anderson (Alyson Publications, 2002).

Tantra for the West: A Guide to Personal Freedom, by Marcus Allen (New World Library, 1981).

Tantric Sex, by E. J. Gold and Cybele Gold (Peak Skill Publishing, 1988).

The Tantra Experience, by Osho (Rebel Publishing House, 1994).

Tantric Transformation, by Osho (Rebel Publishing House, 1994).

Videos and DVDs

Ancient Secrets of Sexual Ecstasy. This video presents ecstatic instruction in Tantric and sacred sexuality, appropriate for both beginners and more advanced erotic practitioners. Available from Erospirit at (800) 432-3767 or www.eroticmassage.com.

Annie Sprinkle's Amazing World of Orgasm. Annie Sprinkle presents an eye-gasmic, educational, enlightening, and sexy documentary about the big O, featuring interviews with twenty six orgasm experts, including Barbara Carrellas. Available from www.anniesprinkle.org.

Annie Sprinkle's Herstory of Porn. Annie Sprinkle guides you on a trip to seven different movie theaters, where she interacts with the best (and worst) clips of many of the 150 plus XXX movies that made her a one-of-a-kind star. Available from www.anniesprinkle.org.

The Art of Orgasm: Multi-Orgasmic Couple. This explicit two-DVD program on sexual pleasure is based on Margo Anand's book *The Art of Sexual Magic* and her Multi-Orgasmic Responses Ecstasy (MORE) training workshops. Available from www.margotanand.com.

Celebrating Orgasm: Women's Private Selfloving Sessions. This documentary illustrates Betty Dodson's sex-coaching techniques, guiding women through sexual arousal to enjoying one or more orgasms. Available from Betty's Sex Shop at (866) 877-9676 or www.bettydodson.com.

Evolutionary Masturbation: An Intimate Guide to the Male Orgasm. Joseph Kramer and four personal sex trainers demonstrate over twenty self-erotic massage techniques. Available from Erospirit at (800) 432-3767 or www.eroticmassage.com.

Masturbation Memoirs. Six women, including Annie Sprinkle, discuss and demonstrate their personal masturbation techniques. Available from Erospirit at (800) 432-3767 or www.eroticmassage.com or www.anniesprinkle.org.

The Pain Game. BDSM educator and practitioner Cléo Dubois presents her award-winning S/M video. Scenes include the art of negotiation, light bondage, whipping, erotic pain, play piercing, intense heartfelt connection, and shamanic S/M. Available from www.cleodubois.com.

Rites of Passion. Produced by Candida Royalle, this beautiful, high-quality movie contains two vignettes, one written and directed by Annie Sprinkle, and the other by Veronica Vera. Annie's piece is based on her own experience of discovering Tantra and sacred sex. Starring Jeanna Fine and Nina Hartley. Available from www.anniesprinkle.org.

Secrets of Female Sexual Ecstasy. This educational erotic video features clear instruction and easy-to-learn techniques for awakening, deepening, and increasing the power of female orgasmic energy. It contains footage of Tantric loving, sacred spot massage, and female ejaculations. Available from www.sourcetantra.com.

Selfloving: Portrait of a Women's Sexuality Seminar. This documentary of Betty Dodson's famous Bodysex workshops features ten women, ages twenty-eight to sixty (including Barbara Carrellas), sharing an afternoon of selfloving filled with authentic orgasms. Available from Betty's Sex Shop at (866) 877-9676 or www.bettydodson.com.

The Sluts and Goddesses Video Workshop or How to Be a Sex Goddess in 101 Easy Steps. A feminist porn classic, this video takes a humorous, absurd, heartfelt, and worshipful look at sex, featuring many erotic ways to stimulate sexual and sensual pleasure. It features Barbara Carrellas as a "transformation facilitator." Available from www.anniesprinkle.org.

Tantric Guide to Better Sex/Better Sex Video Series. Nationally recognized experts Margot Anand, Robert Frey, David Ramsdale, Charles and Caroline Muir, and Drs. Carol Queen and Robert Lawrence guide you through Tantric methods and techniques. Available from www.excaliburfilms.com.

Viva la Vulva: Women's Sex Organs Revealed. Ten women pose for their pussy portraits with Betty Dodson, sharing their innermost thoughts about the relationship they have with their genitals. Available from Betty's Sex Shop at (866) 877-9676 or www.bettydodson.com.

MASSAGE

Anal Massage for Relaxation & Pleasure. This video presents two and one-half hours of expert, hands-on demonstration and features the incomparable Chester Mainard, Dr. Carol Queen, and Dr. Robert Lawrence. It's great for all genders and sexual preferences. Available from Erospirit at (800) 432-3767 or www.eroticmassage.com.

The Best of Vulva Massage. This is a video anthology of erotic touch, featuring world-class sex educators, Tantra teachers, erotic bodyworkers, and orgasm coaches. Available from Erospirit at (800) 432-3767 or www.eroticmassage.com.

Fire in the Valley: Female Genital Massage. Annie Sprinkle and Joseph Kramer teach the genital massage strokes featured in chapter 17 of this book, "The Erotic Awakening Massage for People with Pussies." Available from Erospirit at (800) 432-3767 or www.eroticmassage.com.

Fire on the Mountain: Male Genital Massage. Joseph Kramer teaches the joys of giving and receiving the massage featured in chapter 18 of this book, "The Erotic Awakening Massage for People with Penises." Available from Erospirit at (800) 432-3767 or www.eroticmassage.com.

Rosebud Massage. This video features a tutorial in anal massage by the brilliant Chester Mainard, the most well-known teacher of anal massage in the world. Available from Erospirit at (800) 432-3767 or www.eroticmassage.com.

Tantric Massage. This video teaches you how to give a full-body, warm oil, Swedish-Esalen style massage. Available from Erospirit at (800) 432-3767 or www.eroticmassage.com.

Music

DRAMATIC MUSIC

Blade Runner, by Vangelis (Warner Music, 1994).

Odyssey: The Definitive Collection, by Vangelis (Hip-O Records, 2003).

Themes, by Vangelis (Polygram Records, 1989).

ENERGY-BUILDING MUSIC

Aye, by Angelique Kidjo (Island Records, 1994).

Black Ivory Soul, by Angelique Kidjo (Sony, 2002).

Drums of Passion, by Babatunde Olatunji (Sony, 2002).

The Empresses of Africa, by various artists (featuring Angelique Kidjo, Miriam Makeba, and Cesaria Evora and the Mahotella Queens) (Wrasse Records, 2000).

Fifa, by Angelique Kidjo (Island Records, 1996).

Freedom, by Yothu Yindi (Mushroom Records, Australia, 1993).

Lam Toro, by Baaba Mal (Island Records, 1993).

Nomad, by Nomad (Australia Music International, 1994).

Thunderdrums, by Scott Fitzgerald (World Disc Music, 1990).

Tribal Voice, by Yothu Yindi (Mushroom Records, Australia, 1992).

INSPIRATIONAL AND HEART-CENTERED MUSIC

By Heart: Piano Solos, by Jim Brickman (Windham Hill Records, 1995).

Songs from a Secret Garden, by Secret Garden (Polygram, 1996).

Spirited Away (Original Motion Picture Soundtrack), by Joe Hisaishi (Nibariki / TGNDDTM, 2001).

A Taste of Tao, by various artists (Tao Music/New Earth Records, 1992).

Whale Rider (Original Motion Picture Soundtrack), by Lisa Gerrard (4AD Records, 2003).

LATIN BEAT

The Best of the Gipsy Kings, by Gipsy Kings (Nonesuch, 1995).

The Gipsy Kings, by Gipsy Kings (Nonesuch, 1990).

Supernatural, by Santana (BMG/Arista, 1999).

Verve Jazz Masters 13, by Antonio Carlos Jobim (Polygram 1994).

LUSCIOUS LOUNGE MUSIC

Impala Lounge: A Pure Selection of Afro Beats and Electro Tunes, by various artists (Wagaam Music, 2001).

More of Other Worlds, Other Sounds, by Esquivel (Warner Bros., 1995).

Space Age Bachelor Pad Music, by Esquivel (Bar None Records, 1994).

Ultra Lounge, by various artists (Capitol Records, 1996).

MIDDLE EASTERN MUSIC

Any recordings by Sheila Chandra.

Mystic Groove, by various artists (Palm Pictures, 2001; www.quango.com).

Shakti Dancing, by Prem Joshua (White Swan Music, 2001).

Voice of Silence, by Djur Djura (Luaka Bop, 1993).

MUSIC FOR ACTIVE MEDITATIONS

The Osho Dynamic Meditation, (New Earth Records, 1995).

The Osho Kundalini Meditation, with music by Deuter (New Earth Records, 1995).

MUSIC FOR KEGELS, UNDULATIONS, AND THE WAVE

The Calling, by Kutira and Raphael (Kahua Hawaiian Institute, 1995; www.kahuarecords.com).

Escape, by Mars Lasar (Real Music, 1995).

The Essence of Oceanic Tantra, vol. 2, by Kutira (Kahua Hawaiian Institute, 2003; www.kahuarecords.com).

The Wave, by Kutira (Kahua Hawaiian Institute, 2003; www.kahuarecords.com).

PASSIONATE POP

The Adventures of Priscilla: Queen of the Desert (Original Motion Picture Soundtrack), by various artists (Polydor, 1994).

Erotica, by Madonna (Maverick, 1992).

The Essential Recordings, by Marilyn Monroe (Music Collection International, 1992).

The Language of Life, by Everything But the Girl (Atlantic Records, 1990).

Live & Sleazy, by Village People (Polygram Records, 1979).

PRIMAL/EXOTIC MUSIC

Afro-Desia, by Martin Denny (Liberty Records/Caroline Records, 1995).

Boheme, by Deep Forest (550 Music/Epic/Sony, 1995).

Deep Forest, by Deep Forest (Celine Music/550 Music/Epic, 1992).

The Exciting Sounds of Martin Denny: Exotica/Exotica, vols. 1 and 2 , by Martin Denny (Scamp, 1996).

RELAXING MUSIC

Angels of the Deep, by Raphael (Hearts of Space, 1995).

Like an Endless River, by Kutira and Raphael (Kahua Hawaiian Institute, 1995; www.kahuarecords.com).

Shepherd Moons, by Enya (Reprise/Warner, 1992).

The Spirit of Global Chill Out, by various artists (Flute, 2003).

SEXY SAXOPHONES

Any recordings by Stanley Turrentine.

Late Night Jazz, by various artists (featuring Oscar Peterson, Stan Getz, Charlie Parker, Gerry Mulligan, and Wes Montgomery) (Rebound Records/Polygram, 1995).

Late Night Sax, by various artists (featuring Stan Getz, Gato Barbieri, Charlie Parker, Lester Young, and others) (Polygram, 1996).

SOULFULLY SEXY SOUNDS

Any recordings by Aretha Franklin or Tina Turner.

Barry White's Greatest Hits, by Barry White (Casablanca Records, 1975).

Every Great Motown Hit of Marvin Gaye, by Marvin Gaye (Motown, 1983).

Real Love, by Lisa Stansfield (Arista, 1991).

SOUND COLLAGES/ELECTRONICA

The Cross of Changes, by Enigma (Charisma Records, 1993).

The Eleventh Hour, by Mars Lasar (Real Music, 1993).

MCMXC A.D., by Enigma (Virgin Records, 1990).

Moodfood, by Moodswings (Arista, 1992).

Voyageur, by Enigma (Virgin Music, 2003).

SOUNDS OF SPACE

Galaxies, by Kevin Braheny (Hearts of Space, 1988).

Star Trek: The Voyage Home (Original Motion Picture Soundtrack), by Leonard Rosenman (Paramount Pictures, 1986).

SPOKEN WORD

Aural Seductions: Erotic Stories, vol. 1, by Dr. Carol Queen and Fetish Diva Midori (Fire Horse Productions, 2002).

Workshops and Private Sessions

Tantra and sacred sex workshops and their facilitators vary greatly in substance and style. The only way to be sure that a workshop offers what you're looking for *and* welcomes your particular gender, sexual preference, or sexual style is to do your homework. Contact the workshop leader in advance. Ask for references and speak to past participants. When you find the right one, sign up and have a transcendental time!

Barbara Carrellas/Urban Tantra (www.barbaracarrellas.com; www.urbantantra.org)
This book grew out of my Urban Tantra workshops. In turn, writing it all down has helped me create a new line of fun, practical, entertaining, and holistic approaches to conscious sexuality. In my workshops as in this book, I hope to give attendees the benefit of my life experience in Tantra, Tao, metaphysics, performance, ritual, Reiki, rebirthing, commercial sex work, body work, and erotic massage. And like this book, the aim of my workshops is to give participants the experience of conscious and sacred sex, bringing joy and growth to their personal, sexual, and spiritual journeys. All genders and sexual orientations are welcome, but gender-specific workshops are, of course, available.

Margot Anand/SkyDancing Tantra (www.margotanand.com)
Margot Anand, author of *The Art of Sexual Ecstasy* and *The Art of Sexual Magic*, teaches Tantra workshops worldwide. Her SkyDancing Tantra methods combine Tantric, Taoist, and American Indian traditions with the modern techniques of bioenergetics, NLP, sacred ritual, sexual magic, massage, and meditation.

Art of Being (www.artofbeing.com)
Founded by Alan Lowen, Art of Being offers personal growth workshops and seminars that promote awareness, conscious living, and spiritual and emotional wellness. Alan

Lowen is a wise, creative, experienced facilitator. His Tantra workshops, called Body, Heart & Soul, are highly recommended.

Body Electric (www.bodyelectric.org)
Body Electric is a school of holistic healing arts committed to exploring the healing potential of erotic energy. All sexual orientations are celebrated and all spiritual paths are honored. There are classes for men and women, retreats, special events, and workshops in conscious S/M.

Butterfly Workshops (www.butterflyworkshops.com)
Laurie Handler and other teachers offer workshops, private sessions, and seminars on how to develop a new relationship to sexual energy that accesses a life of love, abundance, and "having it all."

Catherine Carter (email: cathcarter@dodo.com.au)
Catherine Carter, a Transpersonal Counselor and sex therapist in Melbourne, Australia, uses Tantric and Taoist techniques in her private sessions and workshops with women and couples. Workshops include Creating Intimacy and Sensual Harmony Therapy.

Hayley Caspers (email: hayley_caspers@yahoo.com.au)
Hayley's workshops for women focus on "getting what you want." She uses Tantric and Taoist techniques to invite and encourage new ways of experiencing sexuality. Hayley also offers one-on-one coaching sessions to help women get what they want out of a relationship. Hayley is based in Australia, but she travels internationally.

Celebrations of Love (www.celebrationsoflove.com)
This site lists Tantra workshops lead by a variety of instructors.

Cléo Dubois Academy of SM Arts (www.sm-arts.com)
Cléo Dubois and her experienced, highly trained staff offer Erotic Dominance workshops for men and women, as well as personalized instruction and private coaching in the BDSM arts for adventurous couples and singles of all sexual persuasions.

Dark Odyssey (www.darkodyssey.com)
Dark Odyssey is a weekend convention that brings together sexuality, spirituality, education, and play in a fun, supportive, diverse environment.

Domina Reform School (www.dominareformschool.com)
Mistress J, a delightful and highly entertaining dominatrix, gives workshops on sex and conscious S/M in Sydney and Melbourne, Australia. She is also the author of *Private Theatre: Personal Observations and Revelations of a Dominatrix.*

LaSara Firefox (www.lasara.us)
LaSara is a sex-positive, poly, bi, Pagan author who has been writing about sexuality and spirituality for over a decade. She designs and facilitates workshops on topics related to both.

Jade Goddess (www.jadegoddess.com)

Saida Desilets offers Taoist-based workshops for men and women internationally. Jade Goddess is an intensive program dedicated to the education and empowerment of sexual energy as our most potent and creative life force. Taoist yoga and qigong workshops are also available.

The Human Awareness Institute (www.hai.org)

HAI has offered workshops dealing with intimate relationships and human sexuality since 1968. In their words, "We help you define what love, intimacy, and sexuality mean to you, and in turn, how that affects the other areas of your life. There is nothing you must believe, and no allegiance you must pay; no organization to join and no pressure to sell to your friends."

Jwala (www.jwalaji.com)

Jwala, author of *Sacred Sex: Ecstatic Techniques for Empowering Relationships*, teaches workshops and offers private Tantra sessions. She is also a rebirther, masseuse, and sensual clothes designer, offering a line of Tantra-wear clothing.

Kutira and Raphael (www.oceanictantra.com)

Kutira and Raphael offer workshops and retreats in Maui. Their approach to Tantra includes yoga, meditation, breath work, massage, sexual healing, loving rituals, dance, music, theatre, positive ceremonial magic practices, and swims with dolphins.

Mark Michaels and Patricia Johnson (www.tantrapm.com)

Mark Michaels and Patricia Johnson, authors of the books *The Essence of Tantric Sexuality* and *Erotic Empowerment: The Fundamentals of Tantric Sexuality*, offer online and in-person Tantra workshops.

Midori (www.fetishdiva.com)

Midori travels the world lecturing and presenting workshops on a vast array of erotic topics, particularly conscious S/M. She's not to be missed.

Charles and Caroline Muir (www.sourcetantra.com)

Authors of *Tantra: The Art of Conscious Loving*, the Muirs offer weekend introductory workshops and week-long Tantra vacation seminars, as well as books, tapes, and home study courses.

Evalena Rose (www.tantraforwomen.com)

Evalena Rose leads introductory and weekend workshops and retreats for women in Santa Rosa, California. Women of all sexual preferences are welcome, both couples and singles.

Sexological Bodywork (www.sexologicalbodywork.com)

Taught by Joseph Kramer and Chrys Curtis-Frawley (among others), Sexological Bodywork is an intensive course at the Institute for Advanced Study of Human Sexuality, culminating in a Sexological Bodywork Certificate.

Sexy Spirits (www.sexyspirits.com)

Founded by Richard "Anton" Diaz, Sexy Spirits is a sex-positive education center specializing in Tantric and Taoist sexual-cultivation practices. Anton offers weekly lectures, classes, workshops, playshops, and play parties.

Carla Tarantola (www.1tantra.com)

Carla is a Tantra teacher, love coach, and intimacy guide. She offers private sessions and group workshops in New York, Maui, and California.

Online Resources

BDSM

Arizona Power Exchange (www.arizonapowerexchange.org)

The Arizona Power Exchange (APEX) is a support and educational organization for people whose lives or interests include S/M, bondage and discipline, or dominance and submission. This organization promotes safe, sane, and consensual erotic play between adults.

The Eulenspiegel Society (www.tes.org)

The Eulenspiegel Society (TES) is a nonprofit organization that promotes sexual liberation for all adults, especially for people who enjoy consensual S/M.

Greenery Press (www.greenerypress.com)

Greenery Press publishes many of the best books about BDSM and kinky sex, many with a strong spiritual aspect.

The Society of Janus (www.soj.org)

The Society of Janus is a nonprofit, volunteer-run, San Francisco-based education and support organization devoted to the art of safe, consensual, and nonexploitative power exchange. It's a great site with lots of information.

GLBTQ

Ashram West (www.gaytantra.org)

Ashram West is an ashram for the gay community that teaches Tantra.

QueerNet (www.queernet.org)

QueerNet provides free online services for the gay, lesbian, bisexual, transgendered, queer, questioning and allies, HIV/AIDS, sexual and gender rights, and leather and S/M communities. The site includes mailing lists, websites, and email hosting, and links to all sorts of queer organizations.

Queer Resources Directory (www.qrd.org/qrd)

The Queer Resources Directory contains 25,488 files about everything queer, worldwide.

TantraForGayMen (www.gaytantra.com)

TantraForGayMen is a noncommercial site dedicated to men who love men and who want to learn more about how to deepen their relationship with the Divine through Tantra. It includes a free members/community page.

POLYAMORY AND GROUP EROTICS

alt.polyamory (www.polyamory.org)

This is the home page for the Usenet newsgroup alt.polyamory. It contains resources, links, and FAQs.

Club Relate (www.clubrelate.net)

Club Relate is the masturbation swing club founded by Lynda Gayle and her husband Tom. Club Relate holds its parties in Florida, but the site contains information about masturbation in all its forms, including watching, being watched, helping, talking, listening to others' fantasies, and parties. The site includes a forum for reader correspondence.

Loving More (www.lovemore.com)

Loving More is a national organization and resource center for people who wish to live outside traditional monogamy. The organization also publishes *Loving More* magazine, the only magazine dedicated exclusively to topics involving multipartner relating. The website offers information about polyamory, as well as community resources.

"A Modern Guide to Swinging" (www.sexuality.org/mgswing.html)

This is a very good introductory article about swinging, followed by links for more information.

SEXUALITY AND SEXUAL HEALTH

Adult Industry Medical Health Care Foundation (www.aim-med.org)

The Adult Industry Medical Health Care Foundation, founded by Dr. Sharon Mitchell, features an incomparable list of safer-sex and sexual health links.

The Body (www.thebody.com)

The Body is a very comprehensive HIV/AIDS resource site, featuring 550 topics.

The-Clitoris.com (www.the-clitoris.com)

The-Clitoris.com is a site dedicated to women's sexual pleasure and health.

The-Penis.com (www.the-penis.com)

The-Penis.com is a site dedicated to men's sexuality and sexual health.

Safersex.org (www.safersex.org)

Not just a site about safer sex, Safersex.org also features sex toys and supplies, free speech, pop culture, religion, and sexblogs—a very cool site.

Sexual Health Info Center (www.sexhealth.org/main.shtml)
Initially created as a project by two students at McGill University in Montreal, Canada, the Sexual Health Info Center provides information and forums for adults to discuss human sexuality and its nuances.

Society for Human Sexuality (www.sexuality.org)
This is the Society for Human Sexuality's huge website, devoted to acceptance and understanding of all sexual orientations and all consensual and safe sexual practices. It includes resources, local guides, essays, reviews, and FAQs.

yOni (www.yoni.com)
yOni is an exploration and celebration of the many faces of the Feminine, offering articles on sex, mothering, intuition, menstruation, shamanism, aging, and more. There are interactive discussion forums, an ongoing book list, a sharing circle, and links to a wide variety of other resources for women on the Internet. When you visit the site, be sure to check out www.yoni.com/lover.shtml.

TANTRA, TAO, AND SACRED SEX

Healing Tao USA (www.healingtaousa.com)
Healing Tao USA contains an online store, plus newsletters and a list of teachers certified by Mantak Chia.

The Kama Sutra Temple (www.tantra.org)
The Kama Sutra Temple is a sister site to www.tantra.com.

Nepal Institute (www.newfrontier.com/Nepal)
This site houses the teachings of Swami Nostradamus Virato. It has a good list of references, links, and resources.

Sacred Sex (www.luckymojo.com/sacredsex.html)
This site contains essays and articles by Catherine Yronwode on sacred sex, Tantra, karezza, and other forms of sex worship. This is a personal, noncommercial site.

Shiva Shakti Mandalam (www.religiousworlds.com/mandalam/index.html)
Shiva Shakti Mandalam is an excellent Tantra site from Mike Magee and associates. It has many pages with masses of reliable information, including good graphics, translations of key texts, and lots of Tantra links.

Society for Human Sexuality (www.sexuality.org)
The Society for Human Sexuality is a social and educational organization whose purpose is to promote understanding and appreciation for the many forms of adult intimate relationships and consensual sexual expression. The site is hugely comprehensive and features a section on Tantra.

Tantra.com (www.tantra.com)

Tantra.com is a comprehensive site featuring articles about Tantra, techniques, workshop and teacher listings, personals, and an online store.

Tantraworks (www.tantraworks.com)

Tantraworks is a large, well-maintained site created by Nik Douglas, author of *Sexual Secrets*. It includes an extensive database, links, and a bibliography.

Universal Tao Center Website (www.universaltao.com)

This is Mantak Chia's site; it includes information on Tao and Taoist sexuality, plus a schedule of seminars, retreats, and workshops with Mantak Chia.

TEENS

Coalition for Positive Sexuality (www.positive.org)

The Coalition for Positive Sexuality is a grassroots, direct-action volunteer group formed in the spring of 1992 by high school students and members of ACT UP, Queer Nation, Emergency Clinic Defense Coalition, and No More Nice Girls. The site includes an online forum.

Scarleteen (www.scarleteen.com)

Scarleteen provides information on all aspects of positive sexuality in a stylish, hip, fun manner—a great site.

Teenwire (www.teenwire.com)

Teenwire, Planned Parenthood's award-winning site for teens, provides honest and nonjudgmental information about sexuality, self-esteem, body image, drugs and alcohol, and communication, as well as relationship advice.

YouthResource (www.youthresource.com)

YouthResource is created by and for gay, lesbian, bisexual, transgender, and questioning (GLBTQ) young people thirteen to twenty-four years old. The site offers support, community, resources, and peer-to-peer education about sex and sexual health.

Shopping

Babeland (www.babeland.com)

Babeland is one of the best sex shops anywhere. With retail stores in New York and Seattle, their website is more than just a store. It features a huge reference and sex-help section.

Bliss for Women (www.bliss4women.com.au)

Maureen Matthews's Bliss for Women is Australia's premier sensuality boutique for women and their partners. Located in downtown Melbourne, Bliss's online store ships Australia-wide.

Blowfish (www.blowfish.com)
Blowfish sells sex and sensuality products of every description, from the mild to the wild. Blowfish caters to all genders, persuasions, orientations, and varieties of relationships.

Come As You Are (www.comeasyouare.com)
Canada's first cooperatively-run sex toy, book, and video store approaches sexuality with respect, openness, humor, communication, and responsibility. Come As You Are is service and community oriented, accessible, and disability positive.

Condomania (www.condomania.com)
America's first condom store has grown into a sex shop with lots more than just condoms. However, condoms are still their first priority. Condomania is a good source for TheyFit condoms, the world's first sized-to-fit condom line, with condoms available in fifty-five custom-fit sizes.

Good Vibrations (www.goodvibes.com)
Good Vibrations isn't just a huge online and retail sex shop, but a legendary worker-owned, sex-positive cooperative enterprise, providing all manner and description of sex information, toys, videos, DVDs, books, and community events.

Grand Opening (www.grandopening.com)
Proprietrix Kim Airs runs this creative online sex-positive boutique.

Natural Contours (www.natural-contours.com)
Candida Royalle's ergonomically designed three-speed vibrators are beautiful, quiet, and sexy.

Stormy Leather (www.stormyleather.com)
Stormy Leather is San Francisco's leading manufacturer and retailer of leather lingerie, corsets, street wear, and adult toys. The retail store also hosts classes and art shows.

Versatile Fashions (www.versatile-fashions.com)
Mistress Antoinette's fetish fashion creations include corsets, catsuits, and original designs for all genders, shapes, and sizes.

A Woman's Touch (www.a-womans-touch.com)
This is the website for the sex-positive retail store in Madison, Wisconsin, which focuses on "celebrating romance and sensuality from a woman's perspective."

BODY ADORNMENTS

Body Circle Designs (www.bodycircle.com)
This site sells gorgeous body-piercing jewelry.

Flesh (www.andromeda-nyc.com)
You can find more lovely body jewelry at Flesh's online store.

Tribalectic (www.tribalectic.com)
With over 70,000 items to choose from, Tribalectic's claim that it's "the largest catalog of body jewelry in the universe" certainly could be true.

TwirlyGirl (www.twirlygirl.net)
TwirlyGirl offers fun pasties for all occasions.

People You'll Love to Know

The following visionaries have all brought new levels of consciousness, health, and pleasure to the world. Their sites are filled with passion and wisdom. Many have online shops as well.

Kate Bornstein (www.katebornstein.com)
Kate is a transgender pioneer, performance artist, lecturer, workshop facilitator, and the author of *Gender Outlaw: On Men, Women, and the Rest of Us*; *My Gender Workbook: How to Become a Real Man, a Real Woman, the Real You, or Something Else Entirely*; and *Hello, Cruel World: 101 Alternatives to Suicide for Teens, Freaks & Other Outlaws*. She's the sweetest gender radical I know.

Betty Dodson, PhD (www.bettydodson.com)
The "Mother of Masturbation," Betty is an erotic artist, sex coach, and the author of *Sex for One: The Joy of Selfloving* and *Orgasms for Two: The Joy of Partnersex*. She's a legend.

Ducky Doolittle (www.duckydoolittle.com)
Ducky is a sex educator, writer, and comedian, who began her professional sex career behind the glass at a 42nd Street peepshow. She is funny, touching, and wise.

Louise L. Hay (www.hayhouse.com; www.louisehay.com)
The woman who taught the world to do affirmations also founded Hay House, the premiere publisher of new thought books, audio tapes, and CDs. Louise has single-handedly moved human consciousness forward several evolutionary steps.

Idexa (www.blackandbluetattoo.com)
Idexa performs transformational tattooing in San Francisco.

Jwala (www.jwalaji.com)
Jwala is my first and favorite Tantra teacher.

Joseph Kramer, PhD (www.eroticmassage.com)
The founder of the Body Electric School and the New School of Erotic Touch, Joseph is a visionary erotic bodyworker.

Kutira (www.KahuaInstitute.com)
Kutira is a Tantrika who swims with dolphins, runs workshops, and makes beautiful music in Maui with her partner, composer Raphael.

Linda Montano (www.bobsart.org/montano/index.html)

Linda is a legendary performance artist and one of my favorite teachers. Linda's work investigates the relationship between art and life, with a focus on spiritual energy states. She creates intricate life-altering ceremonies, some of which last for seven or more years.

Fakir Musafar (www.bodyplay.com)

The father of the modern primitive movement, Fakir has explored spirituality in art, body modifications, S/M, primitive body decoration, and rituals for fifty years. He is one of the bravest people on the planet.

Dr. Christiane Northrup (www.drnorthrup.com)

Internationally known for her empowering approach to women's health and wellness, Christine is the author of *Women's Bodies, Women's Wisdom*, *The Wisdom of Menopause*, and *Mother-Daughter Wisdom*. She is wise, warm, and very sex-positive.

Dr. Carol Queen (www.carolqueen.com)

Carol is the funniest, smartest, and sexiest writer, speaker, sex educator, and activist I know. Author of *Exhibitionism for the Shy* and *The Leather Daddy and the Femme*, among many others, Carol is dedicated to making the world safe for sex.

Candida Royalle (www.royalle.com)

Candida is a producer/director of porn films from a women's perspective, the author of *How to Tell a Naked Man What to Do*, and also the creator of the Natural Contours line of vibrators.

Pat Sinatra (www.patstats.com)

Pat is the high priestess of tattooing, located in Kingston, New York.

Annie Sprinkle, PhD (www.anniesprinkle.org)

Annie is the high priestess of sex-as-art and alternative porn. A former prostitute and porn star turned artist, author, performance artist, filmmaker, sexologist, workshop facilitator, and college lecturer, Annie is the ultimate sex-positivist.

Tristan Taormino (www.puckerup.com)

Tristan is one of the brightest and busiest women in sex. The author of *The Ultimate Guide to Anal Sex for Women*, she's also written countless columns, articles, and other books. Tristan also lectures, teaches, directs porn videos, and produces sexy events.

Veronica Vera (www.missvera.com)

Author and founder of Miss Vera's Finishing School for Boys Who Want to Be Girls, Veronica is funny, wise, and ever so stylish.

norrie m⊕y welby (www.cat.org.au/ultra/ultra.html)

Australian "spansexual" activist, norrie works on behalf of transgender and sex workers' health and rights.

Index

About the Author

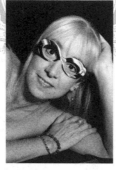

ALLAN PENN

Barbara Carrellas is an author, sex educator, and theater artist. Her pioneering Urban Tantra® workshops were named best in New York City by *TimeOut/New York* magazine. She is also the cofounder of Erotic Awakening, a groundbreaking series of workshops that toured the United States and Australia. Barbara has been featured in several episodes of HBO's *Real Sex.* She is also the author of *Luxurious Loving: Tantric Inspirations for Passion and Pleasure,* numerous articles and essays, and an audio series, *The Pleasure Principle.* Barbara lives in New York City with her partner, trailblazing gender theory author Kate Bornstein.

To learn more about Urban Tantra, visit www.urbantantra.org.